THE
Bloat
Cure

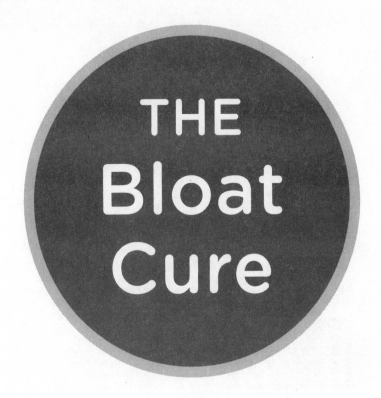

THE Bloat Cure

101 Natural Solutions
for Real and Lasting Relief

Robynne Chutkan, M.D., FASGE

AVERY · an imprint of Penguin Random House · New York

AVERY

an imprint of Penguin Random House LLC
375 Hudson Street
New York, New York 10014

Most Avery books are available at special quantity discounts for bulk
purchase for sales promotions, premiums, fund-raising, and educational needs.
Special books or book excerpts also can be created to fit specific needs.
For details, write SpecialMarkets@penguinrandomhouse.com.

ISBN: 9781583335789

Printed in the United States of America
1   3   5   7   9   10   8   6   4   2

Book design by Gretchen Achilles

Neither the publisher nor the author is engaged in rendering professional advice or services to the individual reader. The ideas, procedures, and suggestions contained in this book are not intended as a substitute for consulting with your physician. All matters regarding your health require medical supervision. Neither the author nor the publisher shall be liable or responsible for any loss or damage allegedly arising from any information or suggestion in this book.

Contents

CONTENTS

CONTENTS

CONTENTS

CONTENTS

Introduction

If you're bloated and looking for solutions, you've come to the right place. In my gastroenterology practice, the Digestive Center for Women, I've helped deflate thousands of women and get them comfortably back into their skinny jeans—and chances are I can do the same for you.

From air swallowing to yeast infections and everything in between, there's always a reason for why you're bloated. Some require just a simple fix, such as switching to a cough medicine that doesn't contain codeine, giving an underactive thyroid a little bloat-busting boost, or identifying a soy allergy that's filling you up with gas. Others are more complex, such as figuring out how to repair a damaged intestinal lining that might be leaking, rebalancing out-of-whack gut bacteria, or speeding up transit time through a sluggish colon. Understanding all the different factors that conspire to bloat you—and having a toolbox of integrative solutions to deal with them—is the key to banishing your bloat for good.

Most of the things that bloat you are benign and fixable, but knowing the signs and symptoms of more worrisome causes that require immediate medical attention is also important. You'll find essential information about those serious sources of bloating here, too.

The good news is you're just a few pages away from identifying the root cause of your bloating. By the time you get to the end of this book, you should be as flat as a pancake. Let's get started!

THE
Bloat
Cure

Acid Blockers

When you think of stomach acid, you probably think of heartburn and ulcers, so getting rid of it may seem like a great idea. But you actually need stomach acid for healthy digestion, and blocking it can lead to serious bloat. Acid helps you break down food and absorb nutrients, and it stimulates your digestive enzymes. It also protects you from harmful bacteria that can enter your body through your mouth. Drugs such as proton pump inhibitors (PPIs) and other types of acid blockers change the pH of your stomach from acid to alkaline, turning it into a nice, friendly place for bacteria to settle and multiply—and produce lots of bloat-causing hydrogen and methane gas.

If you've been taking acid-suppressing drugs for more than a few months, it could be the reason you're bloated, especially if you're having lots of indigestion and gas after eating. It can be easy to confuse these symptoms with acid reflux, though, so you may end up increasing your dose of acid suppression or switching from one acid blocker to another, not realizing that they're the cause rather than the cure.

Solution

- If you're on a PPI, I recommend that you try to go off the drug (check with your doctor first). Taper it slowly to avoid an acid surge, which can happen in the first few weeks after stopping it. Transitioning from daily use to every other day for a week, then every two days for a week, then every three days for a week, and so on, may help you quit more successfully.
- If there's an increase in your symptoms while you're tapering, supplement with shorter-acting antacids if possible, rather than restarting PPIs.
- Elevate the head of your bed by four to six inches with a couple of cinder blocks to make it higher than the foot of the bed, so that gravity can help prevent acid from refluxing up.
- Digestion becomes much less active once the sun sets, so give your stomach a curfew and don't eat after dark.
- Eat small, frequent meals. Your stomach is the size of your fist—overstuffing it will cause reflux in most people.
- Avoid fatty meals, which slow down stomach emptying and increase your chances of reflux.
- Consume caffeine, dairy, and alcohol with caution, since they can worsen reflux symptoms.

Aerophagia

It's normal to swallow a little air when you eat or drink, especially if you're drinking carbonated beverages such as seltzer, beer, soda, or champagne. But as the day progresses, if you feel like the Michelin Woman and fantasize about deflating your stomach with a pin (not a good idea!), you may be swallowing large amounts of air on a regular basis—a condition called aerophagia, which can lead to a massive buildup of gas in your gastrointestinal (GI) tract and major bloating.

Aerophagia is incredibly common but very underdiagnosed, and it's frequently confused with conditions such as ulcers, gallstones, and bacterial overgrowth that can also cause abdominal discomfort and bloating. Most people with aerophagia complain of three main symptoms: bloating, burping, and a tense, distended stomach that feels like an overinflated tire. If you have chronic sinus problems, a deviated septum, or a history of allergies or asthma, you may be a mouth breather rather than nose breather, which predisposes you to aerophagia. Chewing gum, sucking on hard candy, smoking, eating too quickly, talking when you're eating, drinking lots of liquids with your meals, or holding your breath when you're anxious can all cause aerophagia. Eventually most of the air you've swallowed will get burped up or make its way through your GI tract and exit via the other end, but not without causing a lot of bloat in between.

Solution

If you're bloated and think you may have aerophagia, try these tips:

- Spit out the gum and hard candy.
- Eat slowly and mindfully.
- Don't talk on the phone while eating.
- Save drinking liquids for the beginning or end of the meal.
- Drink flat, not bubbly, water and beverages.
- Try some meditation if you feel anxious.
- Practice taking deep breaths that expand your lungs, not your stomach.
- If you're still feeling bloated, a speech pathologist may help you identify whether the problem is related to your speech, swallowing, or breathing patterns.

Alcohol

If you're overindulging on a regular basis, your hangover may come with a side of bloating. Alcohol is toxic to the healthy bacteria in your gut and can destroy large amounts of them, leading to bacterial imbalance (dysbiosis) and bloating. Alcohol can also damage the lining of your stomach, causing an inflammatory condition called gastritis, where the protective mucous layer gets stripped away and acid and digestive enzymes literally start to eat away at your stomach lining, making you look and feel bloated. Alcohol made from gluten-containing grains such as wheat and barley can irritate the lining of your small intestine and cause bloating if you have gluten sensitivity or celiac disease.

Consuming alcohol every day will also add serious pounds to your waistline. It's full of empty calories and gets converted to acetate in the liver, which slows your body's fat-burning processes. Alcohol also dehydrates you, which causes shifts in your electrolytes that bloat your abdomen and give you an overall puffy, swollen appearance. Excessive alcohol damages your liver, leaving you more susceptible to bloat-causing toxins that this amazing organ would normally neutralize.

There are lots of ways to avoid the bloating effects of alcohol without becoming a teetotaler, but if you're drinking every day, it may be time to take a break and see if your bloating clears up along with your hangover.

Solution

- Limit alcohol consumption to no more than one drink a day—less than seven per week (your cancer risk also decreases dramatically below this number).
- Spread out your allotted drinks throughout the week rather than binge-drinking on any given day.
- Drink lots of water in between alcoholic beverages to help flush the alcohol out of your system and prevent dehydration and bloating.
- Safeguard your liver—your main organ of detoxification—by avoiding medications like acetaminophen and tricyclic antidepressants whose side effects include liver damage.

Anatomical Differences

Women may be from Venus and men from Mars, but are our digestive tracts really that different? It turns out they are! Three big differences between the male and female colon explain why bloating is such a problem for us ladies.

The first and most significant difference is that women have longer colons than men—on average four to five inches longer. That may not seem like a lot, but it translates into plenty of extra twists and turns. In medical literature, the twisty-turny female colon is often described as *redundant, tortuous,* or *spastic,* but I prefer to think of it as a *voluptuous Venus colon.* Unfortunately, giving it a nicer name doesn't prevent the products of digestion from getting stuck in all those curves, leading to lots of gas buildup behind the blockage, and plenty of bloating.

The second difference is that women have a wider, deeper pelvis than men. That causes the female colon to drop down into the pelvis, where it competes for space with the uterus, ovaries, Fallopian tubes, and bladder. The result is lots of looping, crowding, constipation, and bloating. Men's reproductive organs take up much less space in their pelvis (their prostate gland is only the size of a walnut), and most of their colon is located above the pelvis in the roomier abdominal cavity, so they're much less likely to suffer from bloating.

The third difference is due to hormone levels: men have higher levels of testosterone, which makes them more muscular overall, including a tighter, more well-developed abdominal wall that keeps their bowels strapped in snugly—sort of like a built-in Spanx. As a result, there's much less tendency for their colon to form loops and protrude. Overweight men may complain of a beer belly, but they rarely complain of being bloated, because underneath all that belly fat is a nice, tight abdominal wall.

If you're constipated and bloated, it may be because you're curvy on the inside: you may be in possession of a voluptuous Venus colon that looks like a Six Flags roller coaster—extra long, with plenty of twists and turns, competing for space with your female parts, and more prone to bulge and bloat because your Spanx is a little stretched out. Fortunately, there are some things you can do to help navigate those turns.

Solution

Being aware of what's going on inside can help you manage your bloat—including figuring out when to lighten up your diet to give your curvy colon a chance to decompress.

- Be careful about eating large amounts of fiber at one sitting, which can contribute to your bloating if your fiber-enhanced bulky stools get stuck in the hairpin turns of your curvy colon. Modify your diet to keep your total fiber intake the same, but spread it out throughout the day.

- Double up your water consumption to help move things through your digestive tract more efficiently and prevent clogs.

- If you feel your bowels getting backed up and you start to become really bloated, do a liquid diet for a day, drinking primarily thin liquids such as water, green veggie juices, and broth to help unclog your pipes.

- On occasion I've had to prescribe a full bowel prep (such as what we use for a colonoscopy) in patients with a stool-filled voluptuous Venus colon. I highly recommend not letting things get to that stage. Do a day or two of liquids if you're feeling really bloated, instead of allowing things to get to the point where you have to blast your bowels.

5

Anismus

Anismus goes by a lot of different aliases: pelvic floor disorder, dyssynergic defecation, inappropriate puborectalis contraction, puborectalis syndrome, paradoxical puborectalis, spastic pelvic floor syndrome, and anal sphincter dyssynergia. But they're all referring to the same thing: pelvic floor muscles that don't relax when you're trying to have a bowel movement. This can make your time on the throne very challenging and lead to lots of backup and bloat. If you suffer from anismus, you may also be experiencing something called *tenesmus*: a feeling of incomplete evacuation. Dehydration and inactivity are risk factors for anismus, but anxiety about bowel movements and holding your stool when you have the urge to go but the conditions aren't ideal are also common causes. Anal fissures that cause pain with bowel movements can also contribute.

If you've been diagnosed with garden-variety constipation and bloating, it's possible that you could actually have anismus. You may have been prescribed laxatives and bulking agents for your symptoms, which generally won't bring relief if the lack of muscle relaxation isn't addressed, too. In fact, if you have undiagnosed anismus, your symptoms may get worse with high doses of fiber, because now you have a big, bulky fiber plug sitting at the end of your colon but your pelvic muscles still aren't relaxing—so you feel even more bloated and uncomfortable.

How can you tell if you have anismus? A test called anorectal manometry can help. It involves inserting a special balloon catheter into your rectum while you perform various maneuvers such as squeezing and pushing. The catheter is connected to a machine that records the pressure associated with these actions and determines whether your pelvic muscles are relaxing appropriately. Defecography is another useful test that provides X-ray images of inserted contrast material as it travels through your rectum and anal canal. It can tell us whether your rectum is emptying properly and identify structural issues such as a rectocele (see "Rectocele," page 154) that may be causing your problem.

Anorectal manometry and defecography are useful tests, but you're probably not in a hurry to have a balloon inflated in your rectum or be X-rayed after being given an enema of contrast material. The good news is that if you have anismus, your doctor may be able to figure it out just from your history and on rectal exam—if you can get yourself to relax enough! During the exam you may be asked to bear down as if you're having a bowel movement. If you have anismus, your doctor should be able to feel your muscles tightening around her finger instead of relaxing. Sometimes just inserting a finger for the rectal exam is challenging because the muscles are so tight, so it may be helpful to do some deep breathing or other relaxation exercises beforehand. Although most people don't look forward to that part of the visit, a good rectal exam can help determine whether anismus is the cause of your bloating.

Solution

One of the most useful strategies for treating anismus is biofeed-back—the process of getting your mind and body in sync. Ano-rectal biofeedback uses an internal sensor placed in the anal canal to record the pressure generated by your pelvic floor muscles. The readings are visually displayed to you via a monitor, and over time, your muscles are trained to respond in a more coordinated manner.

General biofeedback, without an internal sensor, can also help if you have anismus-induced bloating. A belly belt around your waist measures respiration, and sensors on your fingers measure temperature, heart rate, and blood flow. The biofeedback practitioner first gets baseline measurements, and then asks you to think about something stressful to see how your measurements change. Then the real work begins. Using visual imagery, guided meditation, deep breathing, and other relaxation techniques, you're coached to achieve a relaxed state where your breath and heart rate start to sync up, and your muscles begin to relax. The goal is that after a few sessions, you're able to achieve the results on your own without using sensors or a computer, and you can work toward banishing your bloat in the comfort and privacy of your home.

6

Antibiotics

Over the last decade I've witnessed a virtual epidemic of bloating in people who have lots of symptoms but a normal-looking digestive tract. The common thread is often a history of frequent antibiotics. In fact, a detailed accounting of antibiotic use is one of the first things I ask new patients to provide. Some recall being prescribed multiple courses of antibiotics in childhood for strep throat or ear infections; others took tetracycline or doxycycline as teenagers for months or even years for pimply skin; still others received antibiotics later in life for adult acne, recurrent sinus infections, or chronic Lyme disease.

We're only now realizing that the trillions of bacteria that live in and on our bodies—collectively known as the microbiome—play an essential role in keeping us healthy and bloat-free. When you take an antibiotic, you may experience nausea, diarrhea, or vomiting after just a couple of doses. But you may not realize that your long-term bloating could also be a direct result of antibiotics—those you took recently, as well as those from years or even *decades* ago. Antibiotics are supposed to kill pathogens, that is, bad bacteria, but they also indiscriminately kill off huge numbers of the good bacteria that are essential for a healthy gut. Unfriendly fungal species and undesirable gas-producing microbes quickly proliferate to fill the void created by the loss of good bacteria. Even benign bacteria, if their numbers increase too much, can become problematic. The result is *dysbiosis*, a state of bacterial imbalance and one of the most common causes of bloating and GI upset. Lots of factors contribute to dysbiosis (see "Dysbiosis," page 69), but antibiotics are at the top of the list.

You may be like many people who think that simply taking a couple of weeks of a probiotic (live microbes that provide health benefits when consumed) will reverse any damage done by an antibiotic. But just five days of a typical broad-spectrum antibiotic can wipe out a third of your gut bacteria—and there's no guarantee that those missing microbes will ever come back in sufficient quantities. Destroying your gut bacteria with antibiotics and then trying to replace them with probiotics is like draining a full bathtub and refilling it with a single cup of water—literally a drop in the bucket.

The reality is that if you have a healthy, balanced microbiome, you can likely weather the storm of an antibiotic every few years, but you may have a difficult time recovering from excessive use. The drugs are just too potent. And if you've fed your microbes a steady diet of processed food, your ability to bounce back from antibiotics is even more limited, because you likely already have an abnormal ratio of good to bad bacteria that predisposes you to dysbiosis.

Your doctor may have prescribed antibiotics to treat your cystic acne, recurrent sinus infections, or bacterial vaginosis (BV), but that approach is part of the problem, not the solution. Your skin blemishes, sinuses, and vaginal discharge may initially get better, but chances are you'll find yourself in a vicious cycle of recurring symptoms and more antibiotics as your bacterial imbalance worsens. Avoiding unnecessary antibiotics is essential for improving your bloating and can help to clear up these other problems, too, which benefit greatly from a well-balanced microbiome with plenty of healthy bacteria.

Solution

Studies in both children and adults have shown that doctors are far more likely to prescribe an antibiotic when they perceive that the patient is interested in taking one, so there's generally a lot of leeway in whether antibiotic treatment is really needed.

Here are five important questions to ask your health care practitioner if you've been prescribed an antibiotic. The first question is the most important, and while it may not be necessary to go through the entire list, these questions can help frame your conversation and indicate to whomever is doing the prescribing that you're not keen on taking an antibiotic.

1. Is the antibiotic prescribed for me absolutely necessary?
2. Is there an actual culture, swab, or biopsy that shows an infection, or are you treating me presumptively because you think the results will be positive, or to prevent a possible infection?
3. What would be the natural course of my condition if I didn't take an antibiotic?
4. How long should it take for me to start feeling better if I don't take an antibiotic?

5. If I decide not to take an antibiotic, what are the signs to watch for that might suggest that my condition is worsening and I should consider starting an antibiotic?

So you've voiced your desire to avoid antibiotics and queried your health care provider about whether they're absolutely necessary, but the verdict is in: a course of antibiotics is definitely warranted. Now what? Although it's true that your microbiome will take a hit and may be permanently altered, it's still possible to mitigate the damage by supporting your gut and your microbes during and after antibiotics. These ten tips will help minimize microbial loss and encourage rapid regrowth.

1. Take a probiotic during and after antibiotics. Several studies have documented the usefulness of probiotics in decreasing side effects such as antibiotic-associated diarrhea (AAD) and *Clostridium difficile* (*C. diff*; see page 44), as well as repopulating the gut. You should start the probiotic at the same time you start the antibiotic, but try to take the probiotic dose at a time as far away from the antibiotics as possible. So, for example, if you were taking an antibiotic twice daily at 8:00 a.m. and 8:00 p.m., you would take the probiotic at 2:00 p.m. You also need to continue the probiotic for at least one month after finishing the course of antibiotics. Probiotics containing various strains of *Lactobacillus* and *Bifidobacterium* are the most useful, as well as those containing strains of the beneficial yeast *Saccharomyces boulardii* (500 mg daily), which is especially

helpful in preventing *C. diff* and which isn't susceptible to antibiotics.

2. Request a narrow-spectrum antibiotic. Taking a narrow-spectrum antibiotic will minimize damage to your microbiome by targeting a narrower range of bacteria. Culture and sensitivity results from urine, stool, sputum, blood, skin, or other body parts, depending on the type and location of infection, will reveal which bacteria are present and which antibiotics they're sensitive to, allowing your doctor to pick a narrow-spectrum antibiotic that will still be effective, rather than a broad-spectrum one that will needlessly kill off additional health-promoting bacteria. Having the culture results before starting antibiotic therapy ensures that the infection you're being treated for is actually sensitive to the antibiotic you're taking, which will help avoid retreatment with additional courses of antibiotics.

3. Eat prebiotic foods to support your microbiome. Foods high in fiber and resistant starch are especially important when you're taking an antibiotic. Not only do they provide food for your microbes, but they also help to promote species diversity, which can decrease dramatically after a course of antibiotics. Fermented foods such as sauerkraut and kimchi feed your gut bacteria as well as provide additional live microbes themselves.

4. Eliminate sugary, starchy foods. Omitting these foods from your diet is an essential part of creating a healthy

microbiome, and it's particularly important when you're taking an antibiotic. Foods (and drinks) high in sugar and starchy foods that are broken down into simple sugars in the gut send undesirable yeast species into a feeding frenzy, further contributing to microbial imbalance induced by the antibiotics. If you're prone to yeast infections, following a strict anti-yeast diet that excludes any and all sugar while taking antibiotics— and for thirty days afterward—may be advisable.

5. Eat lots of yeast-fighting foods. Antibiotics are the main cause of yeast overgrowth, which can cause vaginal infections and lots of other symptoms. Foods with significant anti-yeast properties include onion, garlic, seaweed, rutabaga, pumpkin seeds, and coconut oil. Make sure you're incorporating lots of these foods into your diet while taking antibiotics.

6. Drink ginger tea. Ginger has a soothing effect on the digestive system and can help to reduce gas and bloating associated with taking an antibiotic. For best results, peel a one-inch piece of fresh gingerroot, cut it into small pieces, and place in a teapot or thermal carafe. Then add two cups of boiling water and let steep for twenty to thirty minutes. Strain and serve.

7. Use bentonite. Medicinal clay has been used as far back as ancient Mesopotamia. Bentonite can help treat AAD by thickening stool, and it also has antibacterial (*E. coli* and *Staphylococcus aureus*) and antifungal (*Candida albicans*) effects. Use one tablespoon of bentonite clay (mixed with water or one tablespoon of unsweetened

applesauce, if desired, for taste) one to two times daily until symptoms of AAD are alleviated. Be sure to separate the clay from the antibiotic and probiotic doses to avoid binding them and reducing their efficacy. Stop using the clay if constipation develops.

8. Make a mushroom tea. Shiitake and maitake mushrooms have been used as medicine by various cultures throughout the world for thousands of years. They have significant immune-boosting properties and antifungal effects. Chop two dried mushroom caps into small pieces. Add them to a small kettle or pot of water (about four cups) and bring to a boil. Reduce heat, cover, and simmer for about thirty minutes. Strain and serve. You can drink this mushroom tea daily while you're taking antibiotics.

9. Support your liver. Antibiotics, like most drugs, are broken down in the liver, so it's important to make sure that your liver is as healthy as possible while taking a course of antibiotics in order to avoid liver damage. Dark green leafy vegetables such as kale, spinach, and collard greens, as well as broccoli, beets, and artichokes, can help keep the liver healthy and promote the production of healthy bile. Avoiding alcohol is essential while on antibiotics, since it increases the likelihood of liver toxicity.

10. Skip the acid suppression. Blocking stomach acid and taking an antibiotic is a recipe for microbial disaster since the lack of stomach acid leaves you vulnerable to overgrowth of pathogenic bacteria such as *C. diff* that

can lead to serious infection. If you think you may require an antibiotic, try to stop any acid-suppressing drugs seventy-two hours beforehand and while taking the antibiotic to allow levels of stomach acid to return to normal.

Appendectomy

For decades, the appendix has been considered an unnecessary organ with no real purpose other than getting inflamed and requiring surgical removal. But it turns out that your appendix plays a very important role: it's where extra good bacteria get stored for when you really need them, such as after an episode of traveler's diarrhea or a viral illness, when your essential gut microbes are really depleted and you're really bloated. Think of it as a microbial reservoir that can help to repopulate your gastrointestinal tract when you're running low on good bacteria.

Solution

Surgeons have a low threshold for whipping out your appendix "just in case," often making the decision to perform an appendectomy (removal of your appendix) during abdominal exploration even if it's not infected or inflamed. That's mostly because of a lack of appreciation for the important role your appendix plays in keeping your gut bacteria balanced. We've seen other examples in medicine where this sort of "just in case" mentality led to poor outcomes—women who were plunged into premature menopause after their reproductive organs were removed because they'd finished having children and their uterus was therefore considered no longer necessary. Just as your uterus has other functions besides making babies (it directs blood flow to your pelvis and genitalia), so, too, your appendix is an important player in keeping you bloat-free. Make sure you don't give yours up without compelling evidence that you'd be better off without it.

8

Artificial Sweeteners

There are lots of good reasons to avoid artificial sweeteners. They're a common cause of bloating because they're not absorbed in the small intestine, and they end up in the colon, where they get fermented by colonic bacteria, resulting in lots of smelly gas. Recent studies also show that these substances are harmful to gut bacteria and can disturb the delicate balance between good and bad bacteria that's an important part of staying bloat-free.

Artificial sweeteners can also increase your insulin levels (a risk factor for diabetes) because insulin is released in response to sweetness, not calories, and artificial sweeteners are plenty sweet. In fact, some studies suggest that diet soda may be an even bigger risk factor for obesity than regular soda, despite the zero calorie advertising. Researchers have consistently found a correlation between drinking diet soda and being overweight. Now, maybe that's because overweight people tend to consume more diet products in an attempt to lose weight. But it also raises the possibility that artificial sweeteners increase insulin levels and create more sugar cravings—because another concern is that artificial sweeteners may condition people to want to eat more bloat-causing sweet foods. Sweetness is an addictive habit, regardless of whether that sweet flavor is from sugar or some other substance. And a lot of the extra weight from too many sweets can end up around your middle, adding actual pounds to your bloat.

Solution

Although I'm an advocate of carefully watching your sugar consumption, when it comes to sweeteners, I always recommend calories over chemicals. As a physician, I'm in favor of technology, but no matter how advanced our science gets, some principles still hold true, and one fundamental is that you can't cheat Mother Nature: sweetness without calories, and without any undesirable side effects? I don't believe it, and the research doesn't bear it out, either. Pass on these edible foodlike substances and choose raw honey instead, even if it comes with a few more calories—you may be surprised to find that your waistline goes down, not up.

Ascites

Ascites is an abnormal buildup of fluid in your abdomen or pelvis that can cause weight gain and a rapidly expanding waistline—it can make you look and feel like you're several months pregnant. Ascites is usually caused by liver disease, but about 10 percent of the time cancer is the culprit (malignant ascites). How can you tell if your bloat is from gas or ascites? When you lie flat on your back, ascites fluid will fall to the sides and accumulate in your flanks, whereas gas will generally sit like a mound on top of your abdomen.

Solution

If you think you may have ascites, you should seek immediate medical attention, because although the causes of ascites are not all related to cancer and many are curable, they're all serious and require an extensive evaluation. In addition to a thorough physical exam, an ultrasound of the liver and abdomen will usually confirm the diagnosis of fluid in your abdomen.

10

Belly Fat

First, the burning question: how can you tell bloating from belly fat? Bloating is usually caused by gas, and it generally ebbs and flows: some mornings you're as flat as a pancake and then by dinnertime you look six months pregnant. Or things are fine for a while and then you have several days when you can't button your pants. For most people, there's lots of variation in their bloating, whereas with belly fat, you never really deflate.

If you're not sure whether your bulge is bloat or belly fat, this may help you figure it out: measure around your waist using a tape measure first thing in the morning and at bedtime every day for several days in a row. If you're bloated, you'll typically see that the number varies quite a bit. If it's belly fat, the measurement shouldn't change by more than an inch.

While you have the measuring tape out, I recommend you use it to find out another super-important number: your waist-to-height ratio, also known as the index of central obesity. I know it sounds very official and a little scary, but you absolutely need to know this number, and here's why: if your waist circumference is more than half your height, even if you're not overweight, you may have more belly fat than you thought, and that could be a real problem.

Having love handles doesn't just determine what sorts of clothes look good on you; it can also predict your likelihood of developing certain diseases. Metabolic syndrome, present in up to 25 percent of Americans, is a deadly combination of risk factors that dramatically increases your chances of developing heart disease, stroke, diabetes, and some types of cancer. Those risk factors include: high blood pressure, high fasting blood sugar, low levels of HDL ("good" cholesterol), elevated triglycerides, and an increased waist circumference.

If you have lots of belly fat, you're more likely to have metabolic syndrome, although it's not the superficial muffin-top belly fat under the skin that's the problem; it's the deeper visceral fat that wraps around your abdominal organs, causing a type of bloating that can be deadly if not addressed.

Solution

If you're tired of having a spare tire around your waist and are concerned about the health consequences of belly fat, here are some tips to help deflate you:

- Pay attention to the quality of what you're eating, which can be even more important than the quantity, especially if your diet includes lots of processed carbohydrates and fats.
- Eliminating carbohydrates altogether is much too extreme and not healthy. Instead, seek out nutritious

carbs from sources such as fruits, vegetables, legumes, nuts, seeds, sweet potatoes, brown rice, and quinoa.

- Control stress. High cortisol levels caused by stress are a major contributor to belly fat.
- Tone and strengthen your abdominal muscles through core exercises rather than just doing cardio workouts.

11

Birth Control Pills

Birth control pills (BCPs) contain various forms of estrogen that can be very bloating. If you're on a high-estrogen BCP, deflating your midsection may be extremely challenging due to fluid and salt retention as well as weight gain. These pills are associated with insulin resistance, a condition that can interfere with your ability to lose weight, especially if you eat a lot of carbohydrates. If you already have a tendency toward insulin resistance or are prediabetic, you may be more likely to become bloated and gain weight from BCPs.

Solution

Weight gain of more than 5 percent of your total body weight after starting BCPs may be a sign of insulin resistance and should prompt a discussion with your doctor about a glucose tolerance test to diagnose it. Using an alternative nonhormonal form of

birth control or choosing a BCP with the lowest amount of estrogen possible makes sense if bloating, weight gain, or insulin resistance is an issue. Ironically, going off BCPs can lead to
temporary bloating and constipation due to ovulation starting
again, especially if you've been on the pill for a long time.

12

Bowel Obstruction

If you're having episodes of severe abdominal pain and bloating that occur suddenly, especially if you also have nausea and vomiting with the episodes, you may be experiencing a bowel obstruction. Obstructions require immediate medical attention to avoid complications such as bowel perforation (a hole in your intestines), which can be fatal.

Most bowel obstructions are caused by scar tissue from previous surgery, but a tumor pressing on your bowels, fibroids, narrowing of your intestines from Crohn's disease, radiation injury, and even severe constipation can all cause obstruction. Obstructions are painful because the bowel above the blocked area stretches as it fills with food and digestive juices. The pain is usually intense and occurs in waves as jam-packed distended loops of bowel try to push their contents through the obstructed area. Sometimes a bowel obstruction develops more slowly and doesn't completely block the passage of stool and air, in which case your pain may not be as severe and may develop gradually but will still cause lots of bloating.

Solution

The most important part of treating a bowel obstruction is coming up with the right diagnosis. A careful history that acknowledges any previous surgery and radiation—even if it was decades ago—as well as any current inflammatory conditions such as Crohn's disease, or mechanical issues such as fibroids or endometriosis, is critical. Weight loss, vaginal or rectal bleeding, or anemia may indicate a tumor.

On physical exam, the backed-up products of digestion can often be felt or palpated, and bowel sounds that signal peristalsis (intestinal contractions) may be absent or abnormally high-pitched. Imaging studies such as X-rays or CAT (computerized axial tomography) scans usually confirm the diagnosis by revealing dilated, air-filled bowel above the blockage. Avoiding food and drink to help decompress the bowel and/or placing a nasogastric tube down the nose to suck out the backed-up intestinal contents usually brings relief. Depending on the severity of the obstruction, surgery is sometimes necessary.

Caffeine

Since caffeine has diuretic properties that help you get rid of excess salt and water through the kidneys, you might think it would help with bloating, but caffeine can actually contribute to your bloat. Its diuretic effect can lead to dehydration, slowing down movement of food through your intestines and causing backups and bloating. Caffeinated beverages, especially coffee, can also overstimulate your digestive system and lead to bloat-causing spasms, as well as worsen some of the conditions associated with bloating, such as stomach ulcers, gastritis, and irritable bowel syndrome.

Solution

There's only one way to do this, and it's not pretty—give up the joe! Going cold turkey will get you there faster, but reducing your intake a little at a time (¼ cup per day) over a few weeks will lead to fewer withdrawal symptoms such as headache, irritability, and sleepiness. There are lots of healthy alternatives to caffeine, including caffeine-free herbal teas, hot water with lemon, green juices, and, of course, just plain water.

Cancer

Most causes of bloating are benign, but compression from cancerous tumors, especially colon, uterine, and ovarian cancer, can fully or partially obstruct your bowels and lead to severe bloating. These cancers usually cause additional symptoms such as weight loss, blood in your stool, severe abdominal pain, vaginal bleeding, or anemia, but sometimes bloating and a change in your bowel habits are the only early signs.

Solution

If you have any concerns at all about whether your bloating may be due to something more serious such as cancer, don't hesitate to seek immediate medical attention. If the first doctor you see isn't taking your symptoms seriously, seek a second or even a third opinion until you're satisfied that cancer has been completely excluded as a cause of your bloating.

15

Candida*

You probably know that yeast overgrowth with fungal organisms such as candida can cause an itchy vaginal discharge, but you may not know that candida may also be the cause of your bloat. When you take antibiotics, large amounts of good bacteria are destroyed along with whatever bad bacteria you're trying to get rid of, and yeast species such as candida quickly overgrow to fill the void. Yeast grows in damp places, such as under your arms, in your groin, in your mouth, and in your gut, where they're involved in fermenting food, a process that produces carbon dioxide gas—and lots of bloat! An overabundance of candida in your intestines can damage the lining of your gut, resulting in poor absorption of nutrients and a condition called leaky gut (see "Leaky Gut," page 118), which is also a major cause of bloating.

Additional signs and symptoms of yeast overgrowth include:

- Depression
- Fatigue

---

* See also "Yeast Overgrowth," page 192.

- Food cravings
- Food sensitivities
- Headaches
- Impaired concentration
- Nail infections
- Rectal itching
- Skin problems such as eczema, acne, hives, athlete's foot, ringworm, and dandruff
- Thrush (white lesions in the mouth)
- Unstable blood sugar

Solution

If you have candida overgrowth, you may be tempted to go on a search-and-destroy mission and treat it with lots of heavy-duty antifungals. But rebalancing your microbiome with essential bacteria that can crowd out candida and keep their growth in check is the hallmark of a successful anti-candida treatment program, not just temporary suppression with medication. Eating lots of indigestible plant fiber to feed your good bacteria, avoiding sugary, starchy foods that attract yeast, and taking a good probiotic can make all the difference for candida-induced bloating.

Carbonated Drinks

Dissolving carbon dioxide in water creates carbonic acid, which gives carbonated water and other fizzy drinks their bubbles and leaves you with a bloated stomach full of gas. Bottled or canned carbonated water often contains sodium and other salts that are added to intentionally enhance the taste—and unintentionally enhance your bloating.

Solution

Choose flat water over fizzy. If you must drink carbonated beverages, leave them open for a while so some of the bubbles escape and they get a little flat before you drink them, or dilute them half-and-half with regular uncarbonated beverages or water.

17

Celiac Disease

If you're bloated and wonder whether there might be a connection between what you're eating and how you're feeling, gluten—a protein found in wheat, rye, and barley—might be that missing link. These days it seems like everyone is on a gluten-free diet, and chances are you know someone who's been diagnosed with celiac disease, an autoimmune digestive disorder that causes damage to the lining of your small intestine as a result of eating gluten.

Celiac disease is still very underdiagnosed, although about 1 percent of the population in the United States suffers from it, and bloating is one of the most common complaints, along with a change in bowel habits (usually diarrhea), fatigue, and malabsorption that can lead to nutrient deficiencies, bone loss, and anemia. If you think you may have celiac disease, it's important to get tested. A screening blood test can check for antibodies to gluten, as well as the genes associated with celiac disease (present in one in four people of European ancestry). If your blood test is positive, then an upper endoscopy that examines and samples tissue from the upper part of your small intestine can confirm the characteristic changes: flattening of the fingerlike projections of the small intestine, called villi, and an increase in white blood cells, called lymphocytes, in the lining.

Solution

Avoiding wheat, rye, and barley may sound pretty straightforward, but if you eat out frequently or buy prepared or packaged foods, it can be a big adjustment. Wheat is used as filler in lots of foods, and barley is often used as a sweetener, so you have to read labels carefully. My advice is to always stick to foods that don't have an ingredient list: fruits, vegetables, nuts, seeds, eggs, potatoes, rice, beans, yams, meat, poultry, fish, and shellfish. It's a great opportunity to eat "close to the ground" by avoiding packaged processed foods, and to discover some new healthy grains such as amaranth, millet, and buckwheat (which, despite the name, doesn't actually contain any wheat). Oats can be problematic if you have celiac disease as they're often processed in facilities that also process wheat, barley, and rye, so there may be contamination with gluten, but if you stick to oats that are certified gluten-free, you shouldn't have any problems.

Consuming lots of gluten-free but nutritionally empty foods is common when you're first diagnosed with celiac disease and are wondering what to eat. Gluten-free junk is still junk, and swapping one refined grain for another can only lead to trouble down the road. People with celiac disease who eat a lot of gluten-free versions of foods that would normally have gluten in them, such as pasta, cookies, bread, and pastries, generally have a much less robust response to their gluten-free diet. Ironically, having celiac disease can have a real survival advantage: forcing you to think about what you're eating, plan your meals carefully, avoid processed packaged foods, and cook more.

18

Chronic Intestinal Pseudo-obstruction

Chronic intestinal pseudo-obstruction, or CIP, comes with all the symptoms of a bowel obstruction—especially bloating— but without any actual blockage. We don't know for sure what causes the gastrointestinal tract to develop so much difficulty pushing the products of digestion through, but damage to intestinal smooth muscle fibers and/or nerves is often present. CIP can be congenital (present at birth) or can develop during adulthood, sometimes as a result of other illnesses.

CIP is a rare disorder, but if you have extreme bloating accompanied by abdominal pain, nausea, vomiting, and constipation, it's worth considering whether this could be the cause of your symptoms. An abdominal X-ray will show the characteristic finding of CIP: air-fluid levels that represent air trapped in loops of bowel above stagnant pools of intestinal fluid, along with dilation of the bowel. If there's no actual blockage, and symptoms have been present for at least six months, then you could have a diagnosis of CIP.

Solution

Dietary changes are the main way to treat CIP, focusing on soft foods and liquids, and limiting fat and solid food, which can slow down bowel emptying. Small, frequent meals (five to six small servings per day) can help to avoid overfilling the intestines and improve CIP-related bloating.

19

Clostridium Difficile

Clostridium difficile, also known as *C. diff*, is a bacterium that can wreak serious havoc in your gastrointestinal tract. It's the cause of one-third of all cases of antibiotic-associated diarrhea and triggers significant bloating and abdominal cramping due to the inflammation it induces in your colon. *C. diff* is widespread in hospitals, where health care workers unwittingly transmit it from patient to patient, leading to colonization rates of up to 50 percent in hospitals and 10 percent in chronic care facilities. About 2 percent of healthy asymptomatic people also harbor *C. diff*, and you may even be colonized with it at birth.

The first step in acquiring *C. diff* infection is alteration of your normal gut flora from antibiotics, which leaves you vulnerable to bacteria such as *C. diff* multiplying. The second step is acquisition, which can occur through contact with a hospitalized patient, health care worker, or asymptomatic carrier. *C. diff* bacteria and their spores are present in feces and can infect you if you touch a contaminated surface and then touch your mouth. After acquisition, the third step is development of disease or asymptomatic colonization. Your age, general level of health, immune status, and medications you're taking all play a role in determining whether you end up sick (acid-suppressing drugs are a major risk factor for developing *C. diff*, since stomach acid is one of your body's main defenses against invading bacteria). If you become infected, *C. diff* proliferates in your gut, releasing toxins that cause severe diarrhea, cramping, and bloating, and in some cases even death. Chronic *C. diff* is increasingly common, and can cause chronic bloating and diarrhea.

Solution

Ironically, our main approach to *C. diff* infection has been to treat it with more antibiotics—and not surprisingly, we're seeing a tremendous increase in the number of infections that are refractory, or resistant, to standard treatment. Resistant *C. diff* has led to a novel type of therapy: fecal transplants that involve transferring stool from healthy donors into the digestive tract of the person infected with *C. diff*. Despite the yuck factor, fecal transplants are currently the most effective therapy for refractory *C. diff*. The best protection from *C. diff* is avoidance of antibiotics whenever possible so that you're less susceptible to being infected, and careful hand washing with soap and water if you've been around someone who may have *C. diff*.

20

Codeine

If you're taking codeine (or other opiate-type drugs) on a regular basis as a cough suppressant, to control diarrhea, or for pain relief, you may be swapping old symptoms for new ones: constipation and bloating. Codeine increases transit time through your gastrointestinal (GI) tract, causing a general slowdown of traffic on your digestive superhighway and, as a result of the delays, lots of bloating. Habitual use of codeine can lead to motility problems in your GI tract and chronic bloating.

Solution

Check to make sure none of the medications you're taking contain codeine or other opiates. If you've been prescribed codeine for pain relief, ask your doctor if there's a non-narcotic pain reliever that might be appropriate instead. Depending on how much codeine you've been taking, you may need to wean yourself off gradually to avoid withdrawal symptoms of agitation, anxiety, nausea, and abdominal cramping.

Colitis

Colitis is inflammation of the colon (the large intestine) and usually refers to a chronic form of inflammation in people with ulcerative colitis. But colitis can also be acute and self-limited, as in the case of infectious colitis. Colitis causes thickening of the wall of the colon and inflammation of the lining, both of which lead to bloating. Bloody diarrhea is the hallmark of ulcerative colitis, although more benign forms of colitis may cause only mild diarrhea and bloating. An inflamed colon is happiest when empty, so meals can be especially problematic, and if you have colitis, you may experience most of your bloating after eating.

Solution

There are lots of effective therapies that can help to heal colitis, including dietary modifications, over-the-counter therapies, and prescription drugs, so it's essential to get diagnosed (usually by means of a colonoscopy) if you think an inflamed colon may be the source of your bloating.

22

Collagenous Colitis*

Collagenous colitis is a form of microscopic colitis that's only visible under the microscope. The inflammation produces a thick band of connective tissue (collagen) just under the surface of your colon lining that interferes with absorption, resulting in loose stools and lots of bloating. Collagenous colitis is more common in women and usually causes episodic diarrhea (but without any blood in the stool), bloating, and weight loss. Nonsteroidal anti-inflammatory drugs (NSAIDs) and acid blockers can precipitate flare-ups, and dietary triggers include dairy, artificial sweeteners, and caffeine.

Solution

If you think your bloating could be due to collagenous colitis and you're having a colonoscopy to evaluate your colon, it's super-important to make sure that several biopsy samples are taken

* See also "Microscopic Colitis," page 133, and "Lymphocytic Colitis," page 124.

from throughout your colon—top to bottom—because the collagen deposits can be patchy and may be missed if only one part of your colon is biopsied. Once the diagnosis is made, avoid NSAIDs and acid blockers, and try eliminating dairy, artificial sweeteners, and caffeine for a few weeks to see if your bloating and diarrhea clear up. Over-the-counter antidiarrheals containing bismuth can help with symptoms, and prescription anti-inflammatory drugs and steroids can also bring relief, but finding out if there's a dietary trigger and then removing it should be the first step.

23

Colonic Inertia/ Dysmotility

Slow transit through your colon, also called colonic inertia or dysmotility, can back things up and lead to lots of bloating. Dietary factors such as not enough fiber or water are common causes of slow transit, and so are medications that slow down peristalsis—or the muscle contractions that move food in your digestive tract—including codeine and other narcotic pain medications, antidepressants, vitamins that contain iron, calcium channel blockers used for treating high blood pressure, and aluminum-containing antacids. It's a long list, so your medicine cabinet is always a good place to look if you're bloated and think slow transit might be the culprit.

Hormonal changes, especially around menopause, and systemic conditions such as an underactive thyroid and diabetes can also contribute to slow transit. Long-term laxative use, especially stimulant laxatives, can lead to a form of colonic inertia where your bowels become sluggish and require increasing doses of laxatives to get relief from bloating.

The best test for diagnosing colonic inertia is a Sitz marker study that involves swallowing a capsule containing about two dozen tiny rings. A few days later, an X-ray of your abdomen is taken to show the position of the rings—typically scattered throughout your colon, consistent with slow transit time through your digestive tract.

Solution

If you've got colonic inertia, there's a lot you can do to help get things moving:

- Drink at least 2 liters of water a day.
- Eat at least 25 to 30 grams of unprocessed fiber spread throughout the day.
- Check your medicine cabinet for any medications that may be slowing down peristalsis.
- Get your thyroid evaluated if you think it may be underactive.
- Stop the laxatives and use a fiber supplement instead, to bulk your stool and move things through more efficiently.
- Exercise regularly to promote peristalsis.

24

Constipation

Constipation is probably the most common cause of bloating, and one of my favorites to treat, because there's almost always a satisfying solution. Since constipation and bloating are so often fellow travelers, treating one usually leads to resolution of the other.

The ancient Egyptians believed that stagnating stool in your colon could result in toxins being absorbed through the lining into your bloodstream, ultimately poisoning your body. If you've ever suffered from serious constipation, you know that a colon full of stool can make you feel poisoned: bloated, sluggish, and toxic. These days, constipation is more common than ever due to our sedentary lifestyle and a diet that's low in fiber and high in processed food, dairy, and meat.

There are lots of different medical criteria for diagnosing constipation. Most are based on stool consistency, whether evacuation is complete, and the number of stools—fewer than three per week being the standard textbook definition. But the fact is that you can have a bowel movement every single day and still be constipated and bloated. I see plenty of patients who move their bowels regularly but always feel full and uncomfortable. When I examine their abdomen, I can feel bowel loops filled with stool like fat sausages. If you're squeezing out a stingy stool every day, you may not even realize you're constipated—and you may be pleasantly surprised when a constipation fix also solves your bloating woes.

There's always at least one explanation—and sometimes three or four—for why you're constipated. Size, shape, consistency, color, ease of passage, and even the odor of your bowel movements are all important clues about why things aren't moving: small pebbly stools might mean diverticulosis; toothpaste-thin ones could be a sign of colon cancer; layered concretions that look like they've been deposited at different times could suggest a problem with contractility of the colon; painful passage with bleeding could indicate a fissure; a foul smell could mean a parasite or bacterial overgrowth (both conditions that typically cause loose stools but can also have the opposite effect). Figuring out the underlying reasons for your constipation and coming up with the right remedy may take a bit of detective work, but when your bowels start to function like a well-oiled machine and your bloating gets banished for good, it's a wonderful feeling.

Solution

Since constipation is a symptom, not a disease, it's always important to get to the root of what's causing the slowdown. It may be multiple things—from diet to lack of exercise to medications to fibroids—so you may need multiple solutions. Here are four of my favorite fixes for constipation:

1. *Take a Fiber Supplement*

Fiber helps create a bigger, bulkier stool that's easier to expel. I recommend using ground psyllium husk—a type of soluble plant fiber—and starting slowly. Think of fiber as a broom that sweeps debris out of your colon and keeps the products of digestion moving through efficiently. Even if you follow a high-fiber diet, you can still benefit from the additional fiber in psyllium (although too large a dose can clog up your bowels and worsen your bloating). Drinking a lot of water with the fiber is essential to prevent it from clumping in the intestines. Start with 1 teaspoon of finely ground psyllium husk once a day in the morning, mixed with at least 8 ounces of liquid and followed by an additional 8-ounce glass of water. You may feel full and even more bloated the first few days, but after a week your body should be used to the increased fiber. After a week, add a second teaspoon in the middle of the day, and after two weeks, add a third teaspoon at bedtime. If you feel better with a smaller dose, go back to just 1 or 2 teaspoons. Be sure to follow each dose with an additional glass of water. If you're bloated, constipated, and also trying to lose a few pounds, daily doses of psyllium can help whittle down your waistline by keeping you full in between meals, relieving constipation, and decreasing your bloat.

2. *Clean Out Your Medicine Cabinet*

Many different medications, both prescription and over-the-counter, can cause or contribute to constipation-induced bloating. Some of the common ones include antidepressants, painkillers, blood pressure medications, vitamins containing iron, and antacids. It's worth looking through your medicine cabinet and checking to see if something you're taking on a regular basis may be constipating you. Ask your doctor or pharmacist if you're not sure.

3. *Develop Good Bathroom Habits*

Every time you ignore the urge to go, you're training your digestive tract to be unresponsive and making your bloating worse. Settling in with the newspaper, getting on your phone, or delving into a good book when you're on the toilet untrains your bowels; these habits send a clear message to your brain and body that you have all day, encouraging sluggish bowel emptying and lots of bloating. But there is hope! You can train your bowels by sitting on the toilet for a few minutes at approximately the same time every morning. Your colon and pelvic muscles will eventually get the message that sitting on the toilet means action.

4. *Change Your Position*

Being in the right position is essential for effective elimination. Squatting is the most natural stance for giving birth and, it turns out, for having a bowel movement, too. A squatting position optimizes the angle of your pelvic muscles and provides gentle pressure on your abdomen from your knees, which helps to push the stool out. Putting your feet on a stack of phone books or (no pun intended) a low stool can achieve the same effect as squatting. If you're flexible, draw your feet up and place them on the toilet seat—but be careful not to fall off!

25

Crohn's Disease*

Crohn's disease, like ulcerative colitis, is a form of inflammatory bowel disease (IBD) that can occur in any part of your gastrointestinal tract and cause all sorts of problems, including narrowing, ulceration, bleeding, and obstruction. Regardless of the location and type of inflammation, bloating tends to be a universal complaint because of the thickening of the bowel wall that occurs. Bloating, decreased appetite, and weight loss may be the only signs of early Crohn's disease, and the lag time between onset of mild, nonspecific symptoms like these and actual diagnosis can be several years, so it's important to keep Crohn's on your radar if you're having major bloating and losing weight, especially if you have a family history of IBD, as about 25 percent of people with Crohn's do.

* See also "Ulcerative Colitis," page 185.

Solution

Diagnosis is often the most challenging aspect of Crohn's disease. X-rays and even colonoscopy may not show the inflammation, which usually occurs at the end of the small intestine (the ileum), an area not within easy reach of the endoscope. More sophisticated imaging techniques such as CAT (computerized axial tomography) scan, MRI (magnetic resonance imaging), or video capsule endoscopy (a tiny ingestible micro-camera in a pill) may be required. Like its sister disease ulcerative colitis, dietary changes, supplements, and more potent prescription drugs all play a role in getting the inflammation—and bloating—associated with Crohn's under control.

26

Cruciferous Vegetables

All gas and bloating is not created equal. Beans and cruciferous vegetables such as cabbage, cauliflower, kale, and broccoli contain potent cancer-fighting compounds and lots of healthy fiber, but they also contain a starch called raffinose that your body can't fully break down and digest. Bacteria in your colon ferment raffinose and produce methane, which you may experience as bloating accompanied by smelly gas. This is what I consider good gas, though, because it's accompanied by the health benefits that eating those foods confer.

Solution

I never recommend completely eliminating the "good gas" foods, because they contain lots of nutrients, but here are some things you can do to cut down on your gas when eating them:

- If you haven't been eating foods such as broccoli, kale, and cauliflower, start with a small amount and gradually increase your serving size to let your body get acclimated to them.

- Add lemon juice to your good-gas veggies to stimulate digestive enzymes.
- Soak dried beans overnight before cooking.
- Avoid canned beans, which tend to cause more gas and may also contain a chemical called bisphenol A in the can lining, which has been linked to cancer and other conditions.
- Cook beans with a sea vegetable such as kombu (found at Asian markets and health food stores), which makes them more digestible because it contains the enzyme needed to break down raffinose.
- Take Beano or Bean-zyme at the start of a meal; both contain a plant-derived enzyme that breaks down raffinose.
- Eat a pinch (about ⅛ teaspoon) of fennel seeds or chew on a stalk of raw fennel at the end of a meal to benefit from its gas-reducing oils. You can also make fennel tea by steeping a teaspoon of crushed seeds or fresh fennel bulbs in a cup of boiling water for ten minutes, or you can add it to salads or cooked dishes.

Dairy*

Dairy is one of the biggest contributors of fat to the American diet, much of it in the form of milk. Lactose intolerance is one of the main reasons I don't recommend dairy if you're bloated or having gastrointestinal issues, regardless of whether the dairy is full cream, skim, or low-fat—but there are additional reasons why your milk, yogurt, or cheese habit may be contributing to your bloat.

We've been pasteurizing milk for well over a hundred years to decrease spoilage from bacteria and extend its shelf life. Pasteurization involves heating the milk to very high temperatures, then rapidly cooling it. The problem is that it also destroys lots of the naturally occurring beneficial bacteria in milk that help to keep you bloat-free. In addition, hormones sometimes given to commercial dairy cows to increase milk production can have an estrogen-like effect, which is a major cause of bloating and can worsen other bloat-causing conditions such as fibroids and endometriosis.

* See also "Lactose Intolerance," page 112.

Solution

Eliminate dairy, including yogurt, cheese, milk, butter, buttermilk, cream, whey products, and ice cream (you may be able to tolerate a little clarified butter or ghee if you're not severely lactose intolerant). Acceptable dairy alternatives include almond milk, coconut milk, rice milk, and hemp milk. Make sure to get the unsweetened and unflavored kind.

28

Dehydration

We don't always pay as much attention to what we're drinking as we do to what we're eating. You may think that as long as you're drinking something, you're hydrating yourself, regardless of what that something is, but if you're drinking "potable bloatables" such as soda, coffee, or caffeinated tea that can have a diuretic effect, you could actually be causing dehydration, which can lead to bloating when dry intestinal contents don't have adequate fluid lubrication to pass easily through your gastrointestinal tract. Not drinking enough water is the most common cause of dehydration, but medications for high blood pressure, antihistamines, and laxatives are also notoriously dehydrating.

Solution

More than half of your body consists of water, and since there are so many factors in daily life that cause dehydration, from medications to caffeine to heaters to air conditioners to simply not enough intake, you need to be sure you're replenishing your body's water supply. Drinking lots of water is one of the best things you can do to banish bloating. It promotes good digestion, keeping your intestines moist and the contents moving briskly, which prevents bloat-causing backups and constipation. I recommend at least a liter a day, although the requirement will vary based on the climate you live in, how hydrating or dehydrating the rest of your diet is, and what your fluid losses are. Start with a liter and increase it if it doesn't seem like enough or if you live in a hot climate. Examining your urine will also help you to assess whether you're getting enough water. Ideally you should be urinating about four to seven times a day, and the color should be a pale yellow, although certain vitamins and medications can give it a more concentrated yellow color.

Keep in mind that the thirst mechanism that sends you in search of hydration doesn't kick in until you're already pretty dehydrated, and by then it can be hard to catch up, so measuring the amount of water you're drinking is a good idea. Paying attention to your liquid intake can be an essential part of banishing your bloat by keeping you well hydrated and your digestive contents moist and moving.

Depression

Most of your body's feel-good hormone, serotonin, is housed in your gastrointestinal (GI) tract, and with depression, both you and your gut may be feeling the effects of suboptimal serotonin levels: sluggish bowels and lots of bloating. Unfortunately, many of the commonly prescribed antidepressant drugs also cause slow transit through your GI tract, so improving your mood with pharmaceuticals may make you even more bloated.

Solution

Opting for "talk therapy" over medication when appropriate and getting regular vigorous exercise may improve both your mood and your bloat. Stress-reducing techniques such as meditation, deep breathing, and guided imagery help to calm your mind and curb your bloat.

Diabetes

Diabetes can affect the nerves that control gut motility and result in a major slowdown of your intestinal contents, causing delayed emptying of the stomach (gastroparesis), or a generalized dysmotility syndrome where it takes a really long time for things to get to the finish line. Both are associated with major bloat.

Solution

The good news is that both gastroparesis- and dysmotility-related bloating caused by diabetes can be improved by controlling your blood sugar through diet or medications.

31

Diverticulosis

Small pockets in your colon that fill with stool—otherwise known as diverticulosis—is one of the most common causes of bloating in people over fifty, and it's increasingly common in younger people, too. Diverticulosis is a result of a diet that's too low in fiber, so it's rampant in more developed countries such as the United States where people eat a diet high in animal protein and fat. The colon has to contract more vigorously to expel the small, hard stool characteristic of a low-fiber diet, which leads to small bulges in the wall of the colon that are frequently referred to as pouches, pockets, or potholes.

Diverticulosis can occur anywhere along the length of your colon, but it's most common in the sigmoid, the part of the colon that works the hardest to push formed stool into the rectum. All that pushing causes the sigmoid to become thickened, as well as full of potholes. Stool can get stuck in these potholes, sometimes for days or even weeks at a time. Having multiple small bowel movements while still feeling constipated is the hallmark of diverticulosis. The longer stool sits in the potholes, the more fermentation by bacteria occurs, producing lots of bloat-causing hydrogen and methane gas.

Solution

In sub-Saharan Africa and other parts of the world where people eat a diet high in unprocessed fiber with lots of root vegetables and legumes, they have large, bulky stools two or three times a day and very low rates of diverticulosis and bloating. In the United States, we recommend eating between 25 and 35 grams of fiber per day, but if you're eating anything resembling the Standard American Diet (what I call the SAD way of eating), you're only getting about 10 grams, and chances are your bloating may be due to diverticulosis.

Fortunately, if you're in the early phases of diverticulosis, dietary improvement—giving the boot to the low-fiber, nutrient-poor diet that may have led to this problem in the first place—can have incredible results. Not all fiber is created equal when it comes to laxation, a fancy term for moving your bowels. Unprocessed, naturally occurring foods such as fruits, vegetables, squash, yams, nuts, seeds, and beans provide us with the type of fiber that has much more bang for the buck than what we get from processed sources such as breakfast cereals, whole wheat bread, fiber bars, chips, and baked goods, no matter what the nutritional label on the package says. Aim for 30 grams of fiber from natural sources: fruits, vegetables, legumes, nuts, seeds, and unprocessed whole grains.

A fiber supplement in the form of 1 or 2 teaspoons of finely ground psyllium husk, mixed with at least 8 ounces of liquid and followed by an additional 8-ounce glass of water can work wonders for alleviating the bloating and incomplete evacuation typical of diverticulosis.

Diverticulitis

Diverticulitis refers to infection or inflammation of your diverticular potholes and is usually accompanied by abdominal pain and tenderness, loss of appetite, fever, and constipation or diarrhea. The longer your stool sits in the diverticular orifices, the greater the risk of developing diverticulitis, so constipation is definitely to be avoided, as are nonsteroidal anti-inflammatory drugs, which increase the risk of inflammation.

Solution

Bouts of diverticulitis can be treated in a number of ways: bowel rest (nothing to eat or drink), a liquid diet, antibiotics (if severe pain, fever, or an elevated white blood cell count are present), and analgesia (pain management). Worst-case scenario includes drainage of any accompanying abscesses or surgery to remove a severely affected area.

33

Dysbiosis*

Microbiome refers to the trillions of microbes that live in harmony in and on our bodies. Dysbiosis is a state of bacterial imbalance within the microbiome, with overgrowth of harmful species and underrepresentation of "good bacteria"—it's also a major cause of bloating that affects millions of people. Why are our microbes so out of whack? There are lots of different reasons, and at the top of the list is the widespread use of antibiotics, not just those prescribed for humans but the large amounts given to some commercially raised animals that can end up in our food.

The prevalence of acid-suppressing drugs and other medications that change the pH of the digestive tract and disrupt bacterial balance is another major cause of dysbiosis and bloating, as is the Western diet, which encourages growth of the wrong type of bacteria in your gut. Too much sugar, fat, and processed carbohydrates can send bad bacteria into a feeding frenzy, leading to an imbalanced microbiome.

* See also "Small Intestinal Bacterial Overgrowth," page 162.

Not eating enough fiber encourages dysbiosis, too. Most Americans only eat about half the recommended 25 to 35 grams of fiber daily, which can negatively affect both the amount and diversity of bacterial species present. Certain types of dietary fiber are what we call prebiotics: non-digestible foods that encourage the growth of beneficial species and are a crucial part of restoring balance when dysbiosis is present.

Dysbiosis doesn't just cause bloating; it's the root cause of many of our modern plagues such as autoimmune diseases, allergies, asthma, obesity, and even some types of cancer. The diagnosis of dysbiosis can be elusive—breath and stool tests are only helpful around 50 percent of the time—and a close look at lifestyle habits and personal history is often the best way to make a diagnosis of dysbiosis.

Solution

It's helpful to have a checklist of risk factors for dysbiosis that can help you identify whether it might be the cause of your bloating. Here are some things to consider:

- Have you taken antibiotics more than four times per year or for longer than two weeks at a time?
- Have you been on birth control pills or hormone replacement therapy in the last five years?
- Have you taken corticosteroids such as prednisone or cortisone for longer than two weeks at a time?
- Have you been on acid-suppressive therapy with proton

pump inhibitors or histamine blockers for more than a month at a time?

- Do you take ibuprofen, aspirin, or other nonsteroidal anti-inflammatory drugs (NSAIDs) regularly?
- When you were growing up, were you a picky eater who rarely ate green vegetables?
- Have you consumed large amounts of sugar and starchy foods?
- Do you drink more than ten alcoholic beverages per week?
- Do you drink one or more sodas or diet sodas daily?

I recommend a three-pronged approach to eradicating dysbiosis that involves *avoidance*, *encouragement*, and *repopulation*.

Avoid medications, foods, and other substances that contribute to the problem, including: acid suppressors, alcohol, antibiotics, artificial sweeteners, birth control pills, hormone replacement therapy, NSAIDs, steroids, and foods high in sugar and fat.

Encourage the growth of good bacteria by consuming foods with prebiotic ingredients that can increase the population of essential gut bacteria, including inulin, a naturally occurring carbohydrate found in plants such as artichokes, chicory, and jicama. Oats, dandelion greens, garlic, leeks, onions, and asparagus also contain prebiotics, especially when consumed raw. Fermented foods, such as sauerkraut, cabbage, and kefir, contribute to the growth of good bacteria and provide live bacteria themselves as a result of the fermentation process.

Repopulate the gut with large amounts of live bacteria in the form of a robust probiotic. Probiotics are live strains of bacteria that can be taken in pill, powder, or liquid form. They aren't considered drugs, so they're not regulated or tested for safety or efficacy, and sometimes marketing can masquerade as science on the various Internet sites that sell them. You may have to do some research to find out which particular type may be best for you, but in general, look for one with at least fifty billion colony-forming units (CFUs) that includes several strains of the two most important groups, *Lactobacilli* and *Bifidobacteria*.

Identifying and remediating the cause of your bacterial imbalance is an essential step in getting rid of your bloating. The three-pronged approach I outlined might take some time before results are apparent, but it offers the possibility of a real cure. If you have severe dysbiosis, rehabilitating your gut flora may take months or even years. Your microbiome wasn't built in a day—it took an entire lifetime. Rebalancing it is a gradual process, but with the right approach, tangible improvements can almost always be made.

34

Eating Disorders

If you're severely restricting calories or purging after meals, your weight may be decreasing but your bloat may be increasing. When protein levels in your blood that reflect your nutritional status fall as a result of insufficient calories, fluid shifts occur to even out the concentration of protein, resulting in fluid moving into surrounding tissues, such as your abdominal cavity. The result is a distended, bloated belly. In addition to the cosmetic disadvantages and the discomfort of bloating, the fluid shifts associated with eating disorders can cause electrolyte disturbances and cardiac abnormalities that can be serious and even fatal.

Solution

Getting professional psychological help is key to taking control of your eating disorder—and your bloating. If your weight is significantly below normal, inpatient treatment may be the safest option.

35

Ectopic Pregnancy

Bloating that occurs with fever, pain, and tenderness in the pelvic area can be a sign of an ectopic pregnancy—a pregnancy that implants and grows in the Fallopian tubes rather than in the uterus. If you have an unrecognized and untreated ectopic pregnancy, you could be at risk for life-threatening tubal rupture.

Solution

If you're having bloating, vaginal bleeding, and lower back or pelvic pain and think you may be pregnant, you should seek immediate medical attention to exclude an ectopic pregnancy. Ectopic pregnancies may terminate on their own, or may require medical or surgical intervention.

36

Endometriosis

Tissue from the uterus present outside your uterine cavity is called endometriosis, and it can be a major source of bloating. Endometrial tissue becomes engorged during the follicular phase of your menstrual cycle, when increasing amounts of estrogen stimulate your uterus to thicken and get ready for possible implantation of a fertilized egg. Endometriosis scattered throughout the pelvis and abdomen also becomes engorged during that part of the cycle, leading to discomfort and bloating. Bits of endometrial tissue can adhere to your bowel wall, causing scar tissue, constipation, and lots of bloating.

Solution

Conservative treatment options including pain medication and/or hormonal treatment are usually tried first to manage symptoms of endometriosis. Surgery that removes as much endometriosis as possible while leaving the uterus and ovaries intact is the next step and is preferable over total hysterectomy, which removes the uterus, cervix, and ovaries, especially if you're thinking of conceiving in the future.

37

Estrogen Dominance

As you approach menopause, your levels of both progesterone and estrogen start to decline, but progesterone decreases more than estrogen, leading to a state of estrogen dominance, a condition highly correlated with bloating. Exposure to xeno-estrogens—compounds produced outside the body that have an estrogen-like effect and create hormonal imbalance in your endocrine and reproductive organs—also contribute to estrogen dominance. Xenoestrogens are widespread in the environment: in hormones given to some commercially raised animals, in pesticides used on produce, and in lots of the plastics and chemicals in everyday use. If you're obese, you may be more likely to experience estrogen dominance because androstenedione, a hormone made in the ovaries and adrenal glands, gets converted to estrogen by fat cells. Birth control pills (BCPs) and hormone replacement therapy (HRT) are also forms of xenoestrogens and a major cause of bloating. Stress can deplete progesterone levels and worsen estrogen dominance.

Solution

Premenstrual syndrome, menstrual disturbances, ovarian cysts, endometriosis (tissue from the uterus present outside the uterine cavity), and fibroids (noncancerous tumors of the uterus that originate from the smooth muscle layer) are all associated with estrogen dominance, and they all cause bloating—so treating estrogen dominance is key in getting bloating under control if you have one of these conditions. How do you treat estrogen dominance?

1. Eat organic produce that hasn't been treated with synthetic pesticides or chemicals.
2. Avoid eating commercially raised animals that have been given hormones.
3. Don't use plastic water bottles.
4. Use gloves when you come into contact with household cleaners and solvents.
5. Consider forms of birth control other than hormonal methods such as BCPs.
6. Think about forgoing HRT (see "Hormone Replacement Therapy," page 102).

38

Fatty Foods

Fat takes longer to digest than protein and carbohydrate, so when receptors in your stomach sense food with a high fat content, they send a signal to the nerves that control stomach emptying to slow down to allow enough time for the fat to be properly digested. That's why even small amounts of fatty foods such as duck breast or bacon are really filling—and bloating.

Solution

Limit your consumption of high-fat foods such as meat, cheese, and cream sauces. If you can't avoid a fatty meal, try to have it earlier in the day when your stomach is more active, instead of at night when digestion is a lot slower and it's more likely to bloat you.

39

Fatty Liver

Fat deposition in the liver is known as hepatic steatosis. Although your liver normally contains some fat (5 to 10 percent), large amounts of fat can be caused by too much alcohol, being overweight, diabetes, high cholesterol, viral hepatitis, some inherited forms of liver disease, medications, and, of course, your diet. We used to think that having a fatty liver wasn't a serious medical problem, but now we know that a large percentage of people with fatty liver go on to develop end-stage liver disease, which can be fatal.

The bloating caused by fatty liver won't kill you, but if you're bloated and have one or more risk factors for fatty liver, or if you've been told that you have an enlarged liver, it's a good idea to get evaluated (blood work and imaging tests) to see if a fatty liver could be pressing on your bowels and making you bloated.

Solution

Most of the medications used to treat fatty liver have undesirable side effects, including an increase in heart attacks or weight gain, or just aren't effective enough. What does work to reduce both fat in your liver and your bloat is a radical change in your diet: more green leafy vegetables, legumes, and other plants, and less animal protein and starchy, sugary food. Best of all, that change comes with desirable side effects such as weight loss, a decrease in heart attacks, a healthier liver—and less bloat!

Fibroids

Fibroids are noncancerous tumors that begin in the smooth muscle layer of your uterus. If you have multiple fibroids—as many women do—or a single large fibroid, your uterus may get big enough to squish your bowels and cause major bloating. Fibroids are also associated with high levels of estrogens (see "Estrogen Dominance," page 77), which can also make your bloating worse.

Solution

Fibroids tend to shrink after menopause, when hormone levels decline, so if you're getting close, watchful waiting may be the best option. Drugs that induce menopause by blocking hormone production can also shrink fibroids but can't be used for more than a few months because they cause bone loss, too. Cutting off the blood supply (uterine artery embolization) by inserting small coils into the blood vessels that feed the fibroids, surgical re-moval (myomectomy), or a hysterectomy to take out the entire uterus are all options, depending on the severity of the fibroids, but keep in mind that scar tissue that occurs after a hysterectomy can also lead to bloating.

41

Fructose Malabsorption

Fructose is a simple sugar that's normally absorbed directly into the bloodstream from the small intestine. Most people can absorb about 50 grams of fructose with each meal, but if you have fructose malabsorption, you're able to absorb only half that amount. Unabsorbed fructose ends up in your large intestine (colon), where it gets fermented by gut bacteria, and in the process produces lots of bloat-causing hydrogen, methane, and carbon dioxide gases. As if that's not bad enough, excessive fructose consumption can also lead to bacterial overgrowth, problems with candida, and weight gain—all of which make bloating a lot worse.

Solution

If you think you might be one of the 30 percent of the population that has fructose malabsorption, stick to 25 grams or less of daily fructose. Choose more natural sources of fructose, such as fresh fruits and vegetables, overprocessed food and soda, which contain high fructose corn syrup and don't have any nutritional value. Be on the lookout for unexpected sources of fructose, such as applesauce, dried fruits, cereal, fruit juices, and salad dressings.

42

Gallbladder Problems

Your gallbladder is located under your rib cage on the right side of your abdomen, just below your liver. It's a small sac about the size and shape of a pear, and its main job is to store and release bile. Bile helps with the absorption of fat by emulsifying it—basically mixing it with the watery secretions of your intestines, similar to how dishwashing liquid helps dissolve grease on plates. Too much fat in your diet can cause gallbladder problems, including gallstones (cholelithiasis), poor function (cholecystopathy), and infection (cholecystitis).

All different types of gallbladder problems can lead to bloating, although you may be surprised to know that the most common cause of gallbladder-related bloating is unnecessary removal of your gallbladder! More than half of people with gallstones are asymptomatic, but many of them are advised to have their gallbladder removed anyway, "just in case." In the absence of a clear need for surgery such as acute infection or blockage of your bile ducts by gallstones, it's a good idea to try to hold on to your gallbladder. Here's why: symptoms such as bloating, abdominal discomfort, and nausea may not be resolved by simply taking out your gallbladder. Even when it's functioning poorly and causing those symptoms, removing it doesn't address the fundamental problem behind why it's not working, which is usually a diet too high in fat and processed carbohydrates. Without the gallbladder to store and secrete just the right amount of bile after meals, there's either too much or not enough bile being circulated. Severe bloating after eating is what most people complain of after having their gallbladder out, and some also report diarrhea, nausea, abdominal pain, and malabsorption—lots of reasons to think twice before going under the knife.

Solution

If you thought you had problems with bloating before your gallbladder was removed, you may have even more difficulty after. Removing your gallbladder without changing your diet is unlikely to make your bloating go away; almost 25 percent of people have recurrence of symptoms after their gallbladder is removed. Try changing your diet instead—swap animal products such as meat and dairy for plants, and keep an eye on your fat intake. Your gallbladder—and your bloat—will thank you.

43

Gastroparesis

Everyone with gastroparesis—delayed emptying of the stomach—complains of bloating. We don't know the specific cause of gastroparesis in most people, although there are lots of different reasons it can develop. The vagus nerve, which controls stomach emptying, can be damaged or affected by illness, causing the muscles to not work properly. Diabetes, intestinal surgery, narcotic medications, certain antidepressants, and neurological conditions such as Parkinson's disease and multiple sclerosis are also causes, and gastroparesis can occur after some viral illnesses.

Symptoms can be severe, especially in diabetics, whose stomach emptying can completely shut down if their blood sugar is poorly controlled, leading to pain, bloating, and recurrent episodes of vomiting after eating. Fortunately, gastroparesis symptoms are much less severe in most people and usually fluctuate, with flare-ups that can be precipitated by a large fatty meal or by filling up on too much fiber in one sitting.

If you have gastroparesis, you're probably experiencing bloating, abdominal pain, and feeling very full after eating, especially with fatty meals. Fat takes longer to digest than other kinds of food, so when receptors in the stomach sense a high fat content, they send a signal to the nerves that control stomach emptying to slow down even more, making your gastroparesis worse.

Solution

You might be tempted to skip meals if you have gastroparesis, which turns out to be a bad idea, because it invariably results in overeating later in the day when your stomach is even less active. Eat small, frequent meals instead. Your stomach is only about the size of your fist. It can be stretched to a much larger capacity, but not without causing lots of bloating. Instead of a large or even normal-sized meal, eat mini-meals every three to four hours that will keep you from getting hungry while also giving your stomach enough time to empty. You can also take your usual meal and split it into two servings a few hours apart.

One of the most effective strategies for avoiding bloating with gastroparesis is to eat your largest meal early in the day when your stomach is most active, and your smallest meal at night when it's least active (see "Late-Night Eating," page 114). Waiting three to four hours after eating before exercising vigorously or lying down will ensure you're not jogging or sleeping with a full stomach, although a brisk walk after meals will encourage peristalsis and help get rid of bloating. From a dietary standpoint, if you have gastroparesis, it's important to limit foods with a high fat content, such as meat, cheese, and cream sauces, which slow down stomach emptying even more. You may also need to split up your fiber consumption to avoid overfilling your stomach. Hydration is important for moving things through your gastro-intestinal tract, but chugging large amounts of fluid at one time can make you extra bloated and uncomfortable, and carbonated beverages are definitely to be avoided. Sip on fluids throughout the day instead, and drink liquids in between rather than during meals to avoid additional bloat.

Genetically
Modified Food

Genetic modification involves taking the genetic material from one organism and inserting it into the genetic code of another, creating new substances such as potatoes with bacteria genes, pigs with human genes, and fish with cattle genes. More than 70 percent of processed foods on supermarket shelves today contain genetically modified ingredients.

Potential benefits of genetic modification include enhanced nutrient content, improved taste, resistance to pathogens and disease, enhanced shelf life, and food that's generally cheaper to grow. The downside is that nature is an incredibly complex system of interconnected species, and many scientists worry about the long-term risks, as well as unintended and irreversible consequences, of tampering with that process. Your bloating just might be one of those consequences. Several chronic digestive complaints have popped up since the mainstream introduction of genetically modified foods in the late 1990s. The biggest increase is in the area of food allergies, food intolerances, and microscopic inflammation in the gut—all of which cause bloating.

Solution

In 2010, the American Academy of Environmental Medicine recommended that physicians tell their patients to exclude genetically modified foods from their diets. Like many other organizations, it also called for more independent, long-term safety studies and the labeling of foods that contain genetically modified ingredients. We're still learning about the long-term effects of genetic modification of our food. If you're bloated and not sure why, you might consider excluding these foods from your diet (processed foods with lots of ingredients are a good place to start) and seeing whether you get relief from your symptoms—not because there's a clear link, but because there might be.

45

Giardia[*]

One-third of people living in less developed countries and between 2 and 8 percent of people in the more developed world have been infected with giardia. It's one of the most common intestinal parasites affecting humans in the United States. Swallowing giardia cysts in contaminated food or water is the main method of acquiring the infection. Infectious cysts are then excreted in your stool, up to ten billion a day, although only a mere ten or so cysts are needed to cause infection. Transmission is from person to person, or animal to person, with some cases being transmitted from dogs and other pets. Symptoms usually appear a couple of weeks after exposure, and watery diarrhea or soft, greasy stools accompanied by lots of bloating are typical.

* See also "Parasites," page 143.

Solution

Giardia can and often does clear up on its own, but if you're bloated and also have giardia, then treatment with a prescription medication or over-the-counter remedy might be in order. Remember, for most parasites, including giardia, the likelihood of whether they set up shop in your digestive tract and cause symptoms is related in part to how healthy you are. A nourishing diet, lots of rest and exercise, and avoiding chemicals and other toxins are part of creating a healthy immune system and preventing parasites such as giardia from taking hold.

46

Gluten Sensitivity*

Gluten sensitivity, sometimes called non-celiac gluten sensitivity (NCGS) or gluten intolerance, causes symptoms similar to celiac disease when you eat gluten (mostly found in wheat, rye, and barley), and bloating is definitely the most common complaint. Gluten sensitivity isn't considered an autoimmune disease, and there's no damage to the lining of your small intestine. If you imagine a spectrum from normal to severe celiac disease, then gluten sensitivity is somewhere in the middle. It's a diagnosis made on clinical grounds, based on your response to withdrawing gluten from your diet, or reproducing symptoms by reintroducing it, although recent studies have shown that some gluten-sensitive patients may also have positive anti-gliadin antibodies (an immune response produced as a result of exposure to wheat).

In addition to bloating and gas, symptoms outside the gastrointestinal tract, such as brain fog, rashes, behavioral changes, joint pain, and fatigue, are extremely common with gluten sensi-

* See also "Celiac Disease," page 39.

tivity. According to the National Foundation for Celiac Awareness, as many as eighteen million Americans may have NCGS.

Solution

Gluten is mostly found in processed foods, and you need to be aware that replacing those foods with equally processed gluten-free alternatives, which don't have any real nutrients, may also end up bloating you. Instead, stick to whole foods that don't have an ingredient list, such as fruits, vegetables, nuts, seeds, legumes, rice, sweet potatoes, and organic poultry, seafood, meat, and eggs. The good news is that gluten sensitivity is completely self-treatable: removing gluten from your diet will banish your bloat!

47

Helicobacter Pylori

S tomach infection with the bacteria *Helicobacter pylori* is one of the most common infections in the world, and although bloating is one of the most frequent symptoms, most people with *H. pylori* are actually asymptomatic. When symptoms do occur, they can be mild—bloating, heartburn, and nausea; or severe— causing ulcers and even stomach cancer. Acquisition of *H. pylori* increases with age, and although there's some evidence it may not be a problem in children, it could definitely be responsible for your grown-up bloating.

Solution

Helicobacter pylori burrows deep into the mucous layer of your stomach, so it can be a little tricky to get rid of, and a combination of antibiotics is usually required to eradicate it and prevent resistance. Unfortunately, the potent cocktail of antibiotics we use to get rid of *H. pylori* can cause or worsen bloating, so think twice about embarking on treatment if you only have mild symptoms (see "Dysbiosis," page 69, for how to remediate effects of antibiotics if you have to take them).

Hepatitis*

Hepatitis refers to inflammation of the liver, usually caused by infection with hepatitis A, B, C, D, or E virus, or medications that can damage your liver. Acute hepatitis causes jaundice (yellowing of the skin and eyes), flulike symptoms, abdominal pain, and fatigue, but chronic hepatitis can result in major bloating as a result of ascites—an abnormal buildup of fluid in the abdomen or pelvis that can make you look and feel like you're several months pregnant.

Solution

Prescription medications, homeopathic cures, and avoiding alcohol and other liver toxins are all part of the spectrum of treatment for hepatitis. In severe cases where the liver isn't functioning properly, liver transplant may be required.

* See also "Ascites," page 25.

49

High-Fiber Diet

High-fiber foods are good for you and help to increase transit through your gastrointestinal tract, so they're generally a great way to stay regular and avoid bloating. But too large a serving of fiber in one sitting can clog your digestive pipes, causing a backup and major bloat. This is especially true if you're not used to eating a lot of fiber, or if you're not drinking enough water to help move the fiber through your thirty feet of digestive superhighway.

Solution

Consider splitting your fiber intake into smaller servings, and make sure you're drinking lots of water in between. You'll tolerate fiber better if it's eaten earlier in the day when your stomach is active rather than late at night when your digestive tract is literally asleep. Another strategy: go for a brisk walk around the block to help stimulate peristalsis—contraction of your gut muscles—after eating a lot of fiber. Consider replacing more gas-producing forms of fiber such as broccoli and cabbage (see "Cruciferous Vegetables," page 58) with ones that are easier to digest but still good for you, such as zucchini, leafy greens, and carrots.

Hormone Replacement Therapy*

I f you're menopausal and bloated, hormone replacement therapy may seem like the solution, but although it can help alleviate some menopause-related symptoms such as hot flashes, its estrogenic effect usually makes bloating worse (not to mention there are other associated potential health risks, such as cancer, heart disease, stroke, and blood clots). High levels of estrogen also affect where your body distributes fat, causing more deposition of fat in your abdominal area—the last thing you want when you're already bloated!

Solution

Consider more natural ways to alleviate menopausal symptoms, such as plant-derived black cohosh, meditation, acupuncture, and yoga.

* See also "Estrogen Dominance," page 77.

51

Hysterectomy

Women have a longer colon and a more rounded pelvis than men, and the combination causes our colon to drop deep into our pelvis, where it competes for space with our ovaries, Fallopian tubes, uterus, and bladder. This can lead to a lot of looping and bloating. But the situation doesn't get any better if our uterus is removed. Hysterectomy—whether a partial procedure where just the uterus is removed or the full monty where all your reproductive organs come out—leads to formation of scar tissue where the uterus used to be that can press on the bowels and make your bloating even worse.

Solution

If your doctor is recommending a hysterectomy for a benign condition such as fibroids or endometriosis, make sure you've exhausted all nonsurgical treatment options before going under the knife, and keep in mind that these conditions often improve after menopause when there's less hormonal stimulation of the uterus. If a hysterectomy is unavoidable, ask whether your uterus can be removed through your vagina as opposed to cutting open your abdomen, and inquire about leaving in your Fallopian tubes and ovaries, which can all help to minimize post-hysterectomy scarring.

52

Infection

Bloating accompanied by fever can be a sign of serious infection. If your white blood cell count is elevated, too, infection needs to be immediately excluded, particularly from a pelvic, urinary, or gastrointestinal source. Common infections in those areas include pelvic inflammatory disease, cystitis (infection of the bladder), pyelonephritis (infection of the kidneys), appendicitis, gastroenteritis, and ruptured ectopic pregnancy.

Solution

An infection in your abdomen or pelvis will typically cause pain, so the triad of fever, abdominal or pelvic pain, and bloating is particularly worrisome and warrants immediate medical attention to rule out a serious infection or, in the case of an ectopic pregnancy, a potentially life-threatening situation.

53

Inflammation

Inflammation is our body's response to something harmful; a protective attempt to stop injury and heal tissue. Because our environment and much of our food contains harmful chemicals, living with inflammation has become a way of life for many of us.

Inflammation isn't always visible to the naked eye, and it can be missed if a thorough and careful approach isn't taken. If you're having an endoscopic evaluation of your digestive tract to evaluate the cause of your bloating, extensive biopsies should be taken throughout your intestines to exclude inflammation. I've encountered lots of people who've suffered from bloating and were told, after a "normal" colonoscopy, that it was all stress-related, only to have the procedure repeated later with biopsies that find significant inflammation.

Solution

Eat the best-quality organic food you can afford to make sure you're not being exposed to synthetic pesticides that could be causing inflammation and bloating. An anti-inflammatory diet that excludes known causes of inflammation—alcohol, refined sugars, processed grains, unhealthy fats such as saturated fat in red meat, and poor-quality animal protein—and focuses on incorporating large amounts of fresh organic fruit and vegetables and healthy fats from nuts and avocados can help heal inflammation and banish your bloat.

54

Interstitial Cystitis

I f you find yourself needing to pee dozens of times a day but expel only a small amount of urine each time, and if you have pelvic pain or pressure over your bladder, plus plenty of bloating, you may be suffering from interstitial cystitis (IC). Like many inflammatory conditions, we don't know what causes IC, but like its sister condition, irritable bowel syndrome, in which the gut is irritable, with IC the bladder is irritable and needs to empty multiple times a day. Damage to the bladder lining that allows toxins in your urine to leak through and irritate it may be part of the problem, and some people have an allergic component to their IC symptoms and notice flare-ups with certain foods or chemical exposures.

Solution

Unfortunately IC is treated with antibiotics far too often, even though there's usually no evidence of an active bladder infection. Frequent antibiotics can lead to overgrowth of harmful gut bacteria in the relatively sterile bladder, and chronic colonization with *E. coli* and other gut microbes can actually worsen your IC-related bloating—so reserving antibiotics for if and when there's an actual infection is an important approach to IC.

Although pharmaceutical remedies such as nonsteroidal anti-inflammatory drugs and antidepressants may help alleviate your bladder symptoms, they come with their own bloat-causing side effects so are best avoided. Pelvic physical therapy, muscle relaxants, and mind-body techniques such as biofeedback, meditation, and massage can help to relax bladder spasms associated with IC, and they have the added benefit of being bloat-busters.

55

Irritable Bowel Syndrome

rritable bowel syndrome (IBS) involves abdominal pain or discomfort that's typically associated with constipation, diarrhea, or both, and virtually everyone with IBS complains of bloating. A full 15 to 20 percent of Americans suffer from IBS, and in addition to being the source of your bloating, it can have a profoundly negative effect on your quality of life.

One of the classic experiments in diagnosing IBS involves inflating a balloon in the rectum. Someone with IBS feels discomfort at a much lower volume of balloon distension compared to someone without IBS. This is the basis for the theory of visceral hypersensitivity—that is, a lower-than-normal threshold for discomfort with stretching and distension of the intestines in IBS, making gas bloat a particular problem. Low-grade inflammation, alterations in the way your gut and brain communicate through the millions of nerve cells in your gastrointestinal tract, and an imbalance between good and bad bacteria (dysbiosis) may also play a role in IBS. Regardless of the particular cause, if you have IBS, chances are bloating is one of your symptoms.

Solution

The cluster of symptoms we call IBS has a variety of causes and triggers, so persistence, patience, and an open mind when it comes to looking for ways to improve it are critical. Although it usually isn't the whole story, stress can be a major contributor to IBS, so finding ways to control it can make a major difference (see "Stress," page 175). Taking an honest and well-informed look at your diet and noticing how small additions of fruits, vegetables, and water can improve things is also important. Finally, steadfastness in searching for a clear diagnosis and making sure that other conditions, such as parasites, celiac disease, and bacterial overgrowth, have been ruled out cannot be overemphasized, since a diagnosis of IBS is often prematurely applied to anyone who complains of bloating.

56

Lactose Intolerance*

Many of us lose our ability to digest dairy products as we age. In fact, more than half the world's population doesn't make enough of the enzyme lactase necessary to break down the lactose sugar in milk. Gas and bloating are classic symptoms of lactose intolerance, but it can be a tricky diagnosis to make because the symptoms overlap with so many other conditions, including irritable bowel syndrome, celiac disease, bacterial overgrowth, and gallstones.

Lactose intolerance is common, but it can also be a sign that you might have other problems that affect the lining of your small intestine and can cause secondary lactose intolerance, such as Crohn's disease or celiac disease. Gastrointestinal infections such as giardia and rotavirus are also common secondary causes of lactose intolerance, which can end up being permanent even after the infection has resolved.

If you're bloated, irrespective of whether or not you have lactose intolerance, you may find that eliminating or cutting back

* See also "Dairy," page 60.

on your dairy intake improves your symptoms. Since there's no compelling reason to consume dairy—you can get plenty of calcium from green vegetables, beans, sesame seeds, and fish, and weight-bearing exercise is a great way to prevent osteoporosis—you don't have anything to lose, except possibly your bloat.

Solution

If you think you may be lactose intolerant but you're not sure, try avoiding any and all dairy for a minimum of two weeks to see if your symptoms improve. You can also do more formal testing involving breath or blood tests. If you're missing the enzyme lactase, then a test dose of lactose will pass undigested into your colon, where bacteria will ferment it into hydrogen that can be detected in a breath test. A blood test that measures the amount of glucose in your blood after drinking a lactose solution is another way to check for lactose intolerance. Failure of your blood sugar to rise indicates your body isn't adequately digesting and absorbing lactose.

Once the diagnosis of lactose intolerance is made, either with a test or by evaluating the effects of removing dairy from your diet, then eliminating dairy products is a great way to control your bloating. Most people have varying degrees of lactose intolerance and can tolerate small amounts of dairy but will have symptoms with larger doses. If your symptoms are mild and you can't live without some dairy, I recommend sticking to occasional small amounts of Greek yogurt and a little aged cheese, which contain less lactose than foods such as ice cream, milk, and mozzarella.

57

Late-Night Eating

You may not realize that your stomach has a bedtime. Its muscular contractions are tied to the light-dark cycle, also known as the circadian rhythm, so it's most active during the day, when the sun is up, and least active at night, after the sun sets—which is unfortunately when you're probably consuming the majority of your calories. To make matters worse, after filling your sleepy stomach with food at night, you may be reclining on your sofa or bed, so you don't have the benefit of gravity and movement to help transport things from north to south. Eating large meals at night is a sure way to feel bloated, and it can also cause or exacerbate acid reflux.

Solution

Calorie shift by eating your largest meal early in the day when your stomach is most active and your smallest meal at night:

breakfast like a queen, lunch like a princess, and dinner like a pauper. Impose a dinner curfew: stop eating at sunset, or shortly thereafter, and if you're going to eat out, make it lunch or brunch rather than dinner, since studies show that people eat much more when they eat out compared to when they eat at home.

58

Laxatives

If you use a lot of laxatives, your colon may become dependent on them over time, especially stimulant laxatives that affect the nerves and muscular contraction of the colon. Prolonged use of powerful laxatives can damage your colon, making it harder to move your bowels on your own, and tolerance often sets in so that you need increasingly higher doses to get the same results. Occasional use of laxatives is okay, but persistently relying on these drugs to get things moving can end up slowing you down even more. If you use a lot of laxatives and find you're still really constipated and bloated, you may have developed colonic inertia, a condition where passage through your colon slows way down, or sometimes even comes to a standstill.

Solution

Retraining your colon how to expel stool on its own, without the stimulant effect of a laxative, can take months (and in some cases even years). The key is to very gradually decrease the amount of laxative you're taking, and slowly increase the amount of indigestible plant fiber and water in your diet. Keep in mind that a slow-moving colon may feel worse with large amounts of fiber or water in it, so go slowly and divide up the doses throughout the day. Sitting on the toilet at the same time every morning, regardless of whether you have the urge to go, is also part of the retraining and will encourage efficient bathroom habits. Small amounts of natural mineral remedies such as magnesium can help soften your stool without any deleterious effects on your colon and can provide a good alternative to laxatives—your gastroenterologist can give you guidance on doses and types.

59

Leaky Gut

Your intestinal lining is like fishing net made of fine mesh with very small holes. Leaky gut, also known as increased intestinal permeability, refers to a condition where the holes in the net get bigger and allow more things to pass through that ordinarily couldn't. While one function of the intestines is nourishment—sending nutrients on their way to all the cells in your body—its other, equally important, function is protection: barring potentially harmful substances from circulating to the rest of your body.

Larger holes in your intestinal net compromise this barrier function, and bacteria, viruses, undigested food particles, and toxic waste products that normally wouldn't gain access to the rest of your body can leak through the intestinal lining into your bloodstream, where they may stimulate your immune system and lead to a wide variety of symptoms, including bloating, cramps, fatigue, food sensitivities, flushing, achy joints, headache, and rashes.

With leaky gut, poor absorption of nutrients can develop as a result of damage to the villi—the fingerlike projections in the small intestine responsible for absorbing nutrients—resulting in deficiencies and malnutrition even if you're eating a relatively healthy diet.

Colon cancer, polyps, gallstones, hepatitis, and ulcers are diagnoses that have been around for a while. They cause changes in the gastrointestinal tract that you can detect with an endoscope, ultrasound, or blood test—you can see and touch them. A diagnosis such as leaky gut is much more nuanced; there's no specific test to diagnose it, and the evidence linking it to things that you can see or touch is murky. As a result, there's a lot of skepticism in the mainstream medical community about the legitimacy of leaky gut as a diagnosis, although opinions are slowly changing as evidence mounts that this is indeed a real and recognizable condition—and a common cause of bloating.

Solution

There's no miracle cure for treating leaky gut, but there are things that can help heal inflammation and restore the integrity of your gut lining. These solutions focus on removing offending agents, replacing good bacteria in the gut, and repairing the damaged intestinal lining.

- Remove refined sugars, dairy, gluten, alcohol, and artificial sweeteners—some of the biggest offenders when it comes to inflammation. Avoid medications such as nonsteroidal anti-inflammatory drugs, antibiotics, steroids, and other agents that can damage the intestinal lining.

- Replace good bacteria with a robust probiotic containing large amounts of health-promoting *Bifidobacterium* and *Lactobacillus* species that can help restore balance in your gut flora. Fill up on green leafy vegetables and other high-fiber foods that help to promote the growth of good bacteria. Fermented foods such as sauerkraut and kimchi can also increase the ratio of good to bad bacteria.

- Repair your gut lining by consuming lots of anti-inflammatory essential omega-3 fatty acids in foods such as fish, flax, hemp, wheat germ, and walnuts. I recommend getting most of your nutrients from real food rather than supplements, but if allergies or the mercury content in fish is a concern, you can take 600 to 1,000 milligrams of a fish-oil supplement containing the omega-3 fatty acid docosahexaenoic acid (DHA). If you don't eat animal products, you can substitute flaxseed oil, chia seeds, and purslane, which contain the plant-based omega-3 alpha-linolenic acid (ALA). Your intestinal-lining cells are avid consumers of glutamine, an amino acid that your cells use as an energy source that has been shown in some studies to help with intestinal injury and may be beneficial in leaky gut. Safe doses in human studies range from 5 grams to about 15 grams daily. Because we're still learning about leaky gut, these treatment recommendations are mostly drawn from anecdotal observation, and most aren't based on rigorous scientific studies. But they're sensible recommendations with a low risk of side effects that can lead to improvements in your bloating and other symptoms if you have increased intestinal permeability.

60

Low-Fiber Diet

As a society, we tend to be overfed but undernourished: 51 percent of the Standard American Diet consists of refined and processed foods, 42 percent is dairy and animal products, and only 7 percent comes from fiber-containing fruits and vegetables. Fiber is like a broom that sweeps the products of digestion through your colon, ensuring maximized bowel movements and minimized bloating. Most of us consume only a fraction of the recommended 25 to 35 grams of daily fiber, and we pay for it in the bathroom. You may think you eat plenty of fiber, but if you're including processed forms of fiber in your tally, chances are you're still plenty bloated and wondering why.

Solution

Not all fiber is created equal: fiber from fruits, vegetables, legumes, nuts, and seeds helps to create big, bloat-relieving stools that are easier to pass, compared to fiber from processed sources such as packaged snacks, cereals, and baked goods. Indigestible plant fiber from vegetables is arguably the most important food for keeping us healthy—and also the most underrepresented in the American diet.

I'm not a fan of counting calories, keeping track of grams of fiber, or anything else that can turn the pleasure of eating into too much of a scientific endeavor, but there is one simple rule I strongly recommend, and that's my 1-2-3 rule: eat at least one vegetable at breakfast, two at lunch, and three at dinner. If you follow this rule, you'll dramatically increase your intake of bloat-busting plant fiber and decrease your risk of heart disease, stroke, and cancer. My own 1-2-3 routine usually includes a smoothie with spinach and berries for breakfast; raw carrots and zucchini with hummus as a snack; and asparagus plus salad with lettuce and tomatoes at dinner.

61

Lymphocytic Colitis*

With lymphocytic colitis, white blood cells called lymphocytes get deposited in the intestinal lining, interfering with absorption and causing episodic diarrhea and bloating. It can be tricky to diagnose lymphocytic colitis because the colon looks normal when it's inspected at colonoscopy, and extensive biopsies have to be taken from throughout the colon to confirm the diagnosis.

Solution

We don't know what causes the increase in lymphocytes in lymphocytic colitis, but triggers for the diarrhea and bloating often include caffeine, artificial sweeteners, and dairy. Eliminating those foods often lead to a real improvement in symptoms.

* See also "Microscopic Colitis," page 133, and "Collagenous Colitis," page 48.

Meat

Diets high in meat and other low-fiber/high-fat foods take longer to digest and can slow down the emptying of your gastrointestinal tract, making you feel bloated and full. Meat also tends to crowd out the healthier stuff, leaving less room on your plate for high-fiber fruits and vegetables that help keep you bloat-free.

When considering whether eating too much meat may be contributing to your bloating, it's also worth considering what your meat is eating: an astounding 80 percent of all antibiotics sold in the United States are fed to animals raised for human consumption, sometimes to treat infections occurring as a result of overcrowding, but more often to promote faster growth. So in addition to slowing down digestion, eating a lot of meat can expose you to unhealthy amounts of antibiotics that throw your gut bacteria out of whack and fill you with gas.

Solution

If you're going to eat animal protein (beef, poultry, wild game, lamb, pork, etc.), it should be organic and grass-fed in order to avoid the antibiotics and chemicals found in a lot of factory-farmed meats and poultry. Limit animal protein to 4 ounces a day (or none at all if you can do without it) and fill the extra room on your plate with plants instead.

63

Megacolon

Megacolon is an abnormal dilation of your colon that can lead to massive bloating. It can be acute or chronic and has a number of different causes, including parasites (Chagas' disease caused by the parasite *Trypanosoma cruzi*), infections (pseudomembranous colitis caused by the bacteria *Clostridium difficile*), congenital abnormalities (Hirschsprung's disease, in which critical nerve cells are absent), inflammation (ulcerative colitis), medications (narcotics that slow down bowel transit), and some neurologic conditions (multiple sclerosis and Parkinson's disease). In addition to severe bloating, if you have a megacolon you're likely suffering from constipation and have abdominal pain and tenderness.

Solution

Bulking agents and dietary modifications may be all that's needed to treat milder forms of megacolon. For acute cases of "toxic megacolon," anti-inflammatory agents such as steroids and/or antibiotics (if infection is suspected) may be necessary. A stool-filled, dilated colon may need to be manually evacuated and then decompressed using a long tube inserted through the rectum that can suck out air. In cases of severe megacolon, surgery may be necessary to prevent spontaneous perforation that can occur when the wall of the colon becomes overly stretched.

64

Menopause

Menopause is associated with fluctuating estrogen levels and falling progesterone levels, both of which can contribute to chronic bloating. There are a couple of important points to keep in mind regarding menopause. The first is that it may occur over a period of several years, with gradual changes in your hormone levels—what we refer to as perimenopause. So you might still be menstruating fairly regularly but having bloating and mood swings and not realize that it's due to the onset of menopause. The second is that the hormonal changes that accompany menopause aren't just limited to your reproductive organs; your entire body is different, including your metabolism and digestive system. After menopause, it may seem as though just looking at food can make you gain weight, and foods that were previously well tolerated may now cause gas and discomfort. Fortunately, menopause doesn't last forever, and neither will your menopause-associated bloating.

Solution

Eating smaller meals with fewer calories, reducing your salt intake, and engaging in regular strenuous exercise are key to preventing weight gain and bloating during menopause. I see so many menopausal women who don't understand why they're bloated and gaining weight, since they've made no changes in their diet and exercise routines. But that's actually precisely why they're having problems—because they haven't made the compensatory changes needed to accommodate their changing hormonal milieu.

65

Menstruation

Despite all the advances in women's rights, there's still a distinct tendency in health care to attribute symptoms in women to stress or anxiety. The very word *hysteria* is derived from the Greek word *hystera*, which means "uterus." We know that women suffer from real diseases, just as men do, and this bias toward ascribing their symptoms to emotions or stress often prevents real problems from being detected early and appropriately treated. That said, it's also true that there can be a hormonal component to symptoms such as bloating, and for a lot of women the common thread is menstruation.

The menstrual cycle is divided into three phases: a follicular phase, followed by ovulation, and then the luteal phase. The follicular phase is defined by increasing amounts of estrogen, which stimulates the lining of the uterus to thicken and follicles (immature eggs) to "ripen" in the ovaries. During ovulation, the dominant follicle in the ovary releases an ovum, or egg, which lives for about a day if it isn't fertilized. In the luteal phase, the remains of the dominant follicle in the ovary, called a corpus luteum, produce large amounts of progesterone, which prime the uterus lining for implantation of a fertilized egg. In the absence of fertilization and implantation, both estrogen and progesterone levels drop, resulting in the uterus shedding its lining—the process of menstruation.

The different phases of menstruation are associated with lots of other changes in your body in addition to what's happening in your uterus: body temperature fluctuations, altered libido, mood swings, changes in thyroid hormone production, neurological symptoms such as migraines, and, of course, bloating. Fluctuating hormone levels lead to an increase in intestinal gas production, an increase in water and salt retention by the kidneys, and a decrease in bile production—all of which worsen bloating. Bile helps to emulsify or break down fats and lubricate the small intestine; low levels lead to accumulation of the products of digestion within the small intestine, causing bloating and constipation. Estrogen is strongly associated with water retention, which is why you may experience bloating in the days leading up to your period as your estrogen levels rise.

Solution

Suppressing ovulation with birth control pills (BCPs) can help with menstrual cramps, but we know that BCPs themselves can lead to bloating, so you're really just swapping one cause of bloat for another. Safe remedies for bloating that occurs every month with your period include a hot-water bottle, chamomile tea, exercise, and acupuncture.

66

Microscopic Colitis

Microscopic colitis is visible only under the microscope and consists of two kinds of inflammation, both of which cause bloating and loose stools: a thick band of connective tissue called collagen under the surface of the colon lining that prevents proper absorption (see "Collagenous Colitis," page 48), or increased deposition of white blood cells called lymphocytes in the lining (see "Lymphocytic Colitis," page 124).

We're not sure what causes microscopic inflammation, but it may be related to long-standing irritation of the gastrointestinal tract. The immune system seems to be responding to something in the gut that's not supposed to be there, and the end result is inflammation, loose stools, and lots of bloating.

Solution

If you're having a colonoscopy to evaluate your bloating, you need to make sure that several biopsy samples are taken from throughout your colon, because the microscopic inflammation can be patchy and might be missed if only one part of your colon is biopsied. Once a diagnosis of microscopic colitis is made, avoid nonsteroidal anti-inflammatory drugs and acid blockers, which can trigger symptoms, and eliminate dairy, artificial sweeteners, and caffeine for a few weeks to see if bloating and diarrhea decrease. Over-the-counter antidiarrheals and prescription drugs can help with symptoms, but investigating whether there's a dietary or lifestyle trigger and then removing it should be tried first.

67

Multiple Sclerosis

M ost people with multiple sclerosis (MS) suffer from bowel problems at some point in their lives, and bloating is one of their main complaints, affecting half of all MS sufferers, and often accompanied by severe constipation. In MS the muscles around your abdomen become weak either due to the disease or because of lack of exercise. Reduced mobility, a decrease in fluid intake, depression, and the effects of prescription medication can also worsen bloating in MS.

Solution

Increasing your water and fiber intake, adding a fiber supplement such as psyllium husk (see "Constipation," page 52), getting more exercise, and training your bowels by sitting on the toilet at the same time every day can all help to alleviate the bloating and constipation caused by MS.

Nonsteroidal Anti-Inflammatory Drugs

Nonsteroidal anti-inflammatory drugs (NSAIDs) may help alleviate inflammation in your joints, but they're a major cause of inflammation in your gut, and they can make you bloated as a result of damage to your intestinal lining. NSAIDs also cause fluid retention, so in addition to feeling bloated, they can make you look puffy all over.

Solution

Look for pain relievers that don't contain ibuprofen or aspirin, and consider an anti-inflammatory diet (see "Inflammation," page 106) or mind-body techniques such as acupuncture and meditation instead of reaching for bloat-causing NSAIDs for aches and pains.

Opiates

Opiates are a class of drugs prescribed to treat pain, but they end up causing bloating and constipation in most people because they significantly slow down movement in your gastrointestinal (GI) tract. Opioid-induced constipation is a well-described phenomenon and a major source of bloating. Infrequent bowel movements, incomplete emptying of your GI tract, hard stools, straining, and bad bloating are all associated with opiate use.

Solution

Pick non-opiate pain relievers whenever possible, and if an opiate is unavoidable, try to take the lowest dose for the shortest amount of time. If you have chronic pain, consider mind-body techniques such as biofeedback, massage, acupuncture, and meditation, which can help manage your symptoms while actually improving your bloat.

70

Ovarian Cancer

Ovarian cancer isn't the most likely cause of your bloating, but it is one of the most lethal. It's only the fifth most common cancer in women, but it causes more deaths than any other reproductive cancer, mostly in women over fifty. Risk factors include never having children or having them late in life, obesity, a family history of ovarian cancer, certain genetic abnormalities, and long-term treatment with hormone replacement therapy. Persistent bloating, feeling full faster than usual, and pelvic pain might indicate a diagnosis of ovarian cancer.

Solution

A thorough pelvic exam or transvaginal ultrasound, where a probe is inserted into your vagina, is the best way to diagnose ovarian cancer. The blood test CA-125 isn't a reliable screening test but can be helpful for following the course of treatment after diagnosis. Ovarian cancer has sometimes been called the silent killer; although it may be that you just have to know what symptoms to listen for—persistent bloating is one.

71

Ovarian Cysts

Ovarian cysts are structures within your ovaries that contain liquid or semisolid material. The most common type of ovarian cyst is a follicular cyst, which forms when the follicle (immature egg) grows larger than normal and doesn't open to release the egg. Follicular cysts usually resolve spontaneously, and any bloating they cause typically ebbs and flows with your menstrual cycle.

Solution

Keeping estrogen levels in check will help to decrease your likelihood of recurrent ovarian cysts. That means forgoing hormone replacement therapy, birth control pills, or other hormonal methods of birth control; eating organic produce that hasn't been treated with synthetic pesticides or chemicals; and avoiding commercially raised animal products treated with hormones. Most ovarian cysts eventually resolve on their own and don't require any therapy, unless malignancy is suspected or they grow very large and rupture, or cause torsion (twisting) of the ovaries.

72

Pancreatic Cancer

This is one of the most dreaded forms of cancer because it tends to be very aggressive and is usually diagnosed when it's already at an advanced, incurable stage, so it has a very poor prognosis. Symptoms are nonspecific but almost always include bloating and weight loss. A significant percentage of people with pancreatic cancer will develop diabetes a few months before their cancer is diagnosed, and blood clots in veins may also occur.

Solution

Fortunately, pancreatic cancer is not a common cause of bloating, but if you do have it, early diagnosis is the key to ensuring a good outcome. Bloating associated with painless jaundice (yellowing of the eyes and skin), weight loss, poor appetite, and upper abdominal pain that radiates to the back may indicate pancreatic cancer and is a worrisome constellation of symptoms that should result in urgent evaluation.

73

Pancreatitis

Pancreatitis refers to inflammation of your pancreas. Acute pancreatitis will usually cause severe abdominal pain and tenderness, nausea, vomiting, sometimes fever, and almost always bloating because of swelling of the pancreas and fluid shifts in the abdomen. Chronic pancreatitis can lead to permanent damage to your pancreas from scar tissue, and extensive scarring may cause your pancreas to stop making its normal amount of digestive enzymes, resulting in trouble digesting food and lots of bloating.

Alcohol abuse is the most common cause of chronic pancreatitis in adults, but gallstones that slip through the gallbladder and block the pancreatic duct are also a common cause (gallstone pancreatitis), as are some prescription medications, including antibiotics, immune-suppressing drugs, antiseizure agents, and diuretics used to control blood pressure. Autoimmune and genetic diseases such as cystic fibrosis can also cause chronic pancreatitis and chronic bloating.

ROBYNNE CHUTKAN, M.D.

Solution

Depending on the cause of your pancreatitis, therapy may include an alcohol treatment program, discontinuation of any offending medications, and/or an endoscopic exam to remove gallstones from the pancreatic duct (and sometimes removal of the gallbladder itself), in addition to bowel rest, pain relief, and IV hydration. Most isolated episodes of acute pancreatitis resolve without complications, but chronic pancreatitis can lead to chronic pain and bloating.

74

Parasites

Parasites can live in your body undetected for years and, in addition to bloating, can create all sorts of problems including diarrhea, rectal itching, blood or mucus in the stool, low-grade fever, body aches, anemia, fatigue, problems absorbing fat, joint pain, teeth grinding, gallbladder dysfunction, and even neurological symptoms. Although many species are harmless and don't cause any symptoms, others can be a major cause of bloating. Three types of parasites can infect your digestive tract: tapeworms, roundworms (also known as nematodes), and protozoa. They range in size from microscopic to several feet long and can stay in your intestines or invade other distant organs.

Parasites are a lot more common than most people realize, affecting a huge number of people worldwide and up to a third of the population in the United States. You may have wondered whether your bloating could be caused by a parasite, even if you've never been anywhere tropical or exotic. The answer is it could be. Common intestinal parasites in the United States include *Enterobius vermicularis* (pinworm), *Giardia lamblia* (giardia), *Ancylostoma duodenale* (Old World hookworm), *Necator americanus* (New World hookworm), and *Entamoeba histolytica* (amebiasis).

Solution

If you think you have a parasite, it's always better to get diagnosed and figure out if you really do, and, if so, which specific one. The treatments can differ dramatically, from single-dose over-the-counter cures to weeks of prescription medication. There are lots of natural remedies, too, including things that may already be in your kitchen, such as garlic, black walnuts, papaya seeds, and cloves. Wormwood tea is effective against many parasites and can be brewed at home, but it's not without potential side effects, including sleep disturbances and, in rare cases, possible organ damage, so it should be used under a doctor's supervision.

In the absence of a diagnosis, beware of signing up for Internet cures that may or may not work and could have unpleasant side effects you hadn't bargained for. You may ultimately need to see an infectious disease specialist or someone with expertise in parasitology. Be sure to ask when you make the appointment if they're familiar with diagnosing and treating parasites.

The good news is even if you're exposed to a parasite, the likelihood of whether it will set up shop in your digestive tract and cause symptoms such as bloating is related in part to how healthy your immune system is. A nourishing and balanced diet is still one of your best defenses for preventing and eliminating these uninvited guests.

Maintaining healthy levels of good bacteria in your gut by

avoiding unnecessary antibiotics and drugs that change the pH will also help to discourage growth of parasites. A high-fiber diet and a daily tablespoon of ground psyllium husk powder can help to remove parasite eggs that may be attempting to make a home. Eating foods rich in vitamin A precursors, such as carrots and sweet potatoes, help prevent parasitic larvae from penetrating, and raw garlic also has antiparasitic qualities.

Parasites can be transmitted from dogs and other pets, so make sure yours are regularly checked for worms and that their feces are properly disposed of. You also need to be on the lookout for whether your pet is eating the infected stool of other animals, a practice that's not uncommon among puppies. To avoid coming into contact with infected stool, don't walk barefoot where animals have been. Strict habits of hand washing, careful washing of fruits and vegetables, filtering your drinking water, and avoiding raw and undercooked meat are also important preventive tactics.

Pelvic Inflammatory Disease

Pelvic inflammatory disease (PID) is caused by infection of the uterine lining, Fallopian tubes, or ovaries, usually from sexually transmitted diseases such as chlamydia or gonorrhea. PID can also occur following childbirth, abortion, miscarriage, or with insertion of an intrauterine device. The localized inflammation causes bloating accompanied by fever, pain, and tenderness in the pelvic area, and a vaginal discharge is very common.

Solution

A careful pelvic exam and treatment with antibiotics are essential for PID, because untreated it can lead to infertility and ectopic pregnancies (pregnancies that implant and grow in the Fallopian tubes rather than in the uterus and, if left untreated, can cause life-threatening tubal rupture). If you're having bloating, vaginal bleeding or discharge, and lower back or pelvic pain and think you may be pregnant, you should seek immediate medical attention to exclude PID.

Polycystic Ovary Syndrome

Polycystic ovary syndrome (PCOS) affects 5 to 10 percent of women of reproductive age and is associated with higher-than-normal levels of male sex hormones (androgens). The classic finding seen on ultrasound is multiple ovarian cysts, and symptoms include excessive facial hair, male-pattern baldness, acne, obesity, irregular menses, decreased fertility, and insulin resistance. Bloating is a common complaint in PCOS, due to abnormal hormone levels as well as the presence of the cysts themselves, which can press on your bowels and cause pain, constipation, and bloating.

Solution

Some studies have raised the possibility that obesity causes PCOS rather than the other way around. What we do know is that addressing obesity and insulin resistance through exercise and a diet that restricts processed carbohydrates such as gluten and refined sugars improves many of the symptoms of PCOS, including bloating. In fact, I've seen high androgen levels, infertility, and irregular menstrual patterns in PCOS resolve with dietary modification and weight loss alone. Classic medical therapy includes birth control pills and hormones to help stimulate ovulation, which are clearly less desirable if you're looking to improve your bloating.

Pregnancy

Pregnancy comes with an expanding waistline that's not always due to just your baby. Rising progesterone levels relax smooth muscle and decrease movement through the gastrointestinal tract, leading to constipation and bloating. The pressure of the expanding uterus on your bowels can instigate a lot of bloat, and even prenatal vitamins can contribute if they contain iron and calcium, which bind things up. Not to mention that many of us are much less active during pregnancy, which slows our bowels and increases our bloat.

Solution

A high-fiber diet, staying well hydrated, and maintaining some degree of safe and appropriate physical activity are essential bloat-busters during pregnancy. Look for prenatal vitamins that contain more natural forms of iron and calcium, which are less constipating and easier on the digestive system. Fortunately, childbirth signals the beginning of a new life and the end of your pregnancy-induced bloating!

78

Processed Food

Over two thousand years ago, Hippocrates, the father of modern medicine, admonished us to "let food be thy medicine and medicine be thy food." It's advice that's perhaps even more relevant today, given the virtual epidemic of digestive complaints we're seeing, in large part due to all the processed food we eat. We've packed our foods with fillers, preservatives, and synthetic vitamins; grow it in an environment full of pesticides and other dangerous chemicals; and have tampered with the genetic identity of the food itself. These modifications are wreaking havoc on our digestive systems, and bloating is our gut's way of signaling its displeasure. My basic definition of food is *something that nourishes you*. Processed foods are anything but—and if you're eating lots of them, chances are you're overfed, undernourished, and plenty bloated.

Procuring and preparing real food is time-consuming, but when it comes to your gut, what you put in is directly reflected in what you get out. Processed foods filled with chemicals will bloat you, no matter what the packaging says about them being all-natural. If I took you into a chemistry lab and told you to open your mouth so I could pour beakers filled with food coloring, 1-methylcyclopropene, monosodium glutamate (MSG), sodium benzoate, sodium nitrite, and other commonly used chemicals into your stomach, you'd be horrified, but that's what you do every day when you eat processed foods.

It's easy to become disconnected from food these days, when so few of us are involved in growing, harvesting, or even cooking the food we eat. But it's impossible to separate what we're eating from how we're feeling, since we truly are what we eat (and what our food eats, too!). Improving your diet doesn't fix all forms of bloating, but it's worth seriously considering whether the food you're eating could be contributing to your digestive problems— a notion that seems intuitive to me as a gastroenterologist but is still not accepted by many in the medical community.

Solution

For this one I'll borrow Michael Pollan's excellent seven-word summation: "Eat food, not too much, mostly plants."

79

Radiation

If you've had radiation to your abdomen or pelvis, you may be experiencing bloating along with more severe symptoms such as abdominal pain and vomiting as a result of either the formation of scar tissue that obstructs your bowel or radiation damage to the bowel itself. Radiation symptoms can occur within a few months of the radiation or years or even decades after, so if you have a history of radiation, even in the distant past, it could be the reason you're bloated, especially if the field of radiation included your abdomen or pelvis.

Solution

If you think your bloating could be the result of radiation, it's important to get a thorough evaluation to exclude an actual blockage (see "Bowel Obstruction," page 31) or tumor (see "Cancer," page 35). If you have milder radiation-induced bloating, eating small mini-meals every three to four hours, drinking lots of water, and getting regular exercise to stimulate peristalsis can all help alleviate symptoms. A clear liquid diet for a day or two and a few doses of an osmotic cathartic can help unclog any more serious backups that might occur from time to time as a result of the radiation.

80

Rectocele

A rectocele is formed when the wall of your rectum bulges against your vagina, which is directly in front of it, as a result of a weakness in the wall between the two organs—usually from long-standing constipation or pressure during a vaginal delivery. Stool can get stuck in a rectocele and cause backup and bloat, and you may have figured out that inserting a finger into your vagina and pressing backward on your rectum can help to get it out. Although this can be embarrassing information to volunteer, it's important to let your doctor know, because if you do this on a regular basis, the cause of your bloat is likely a rectocele or a pelvic floor problem, and there are things that can be done to improve it.

Solution

A radiology test called defecography, in which your rectum is filled with material containing a contrast dye that you're then asked to expel, can show the bulge of a rectocele that fills up with contrast and doesn't empty properly. A high-fiber diet and relax-ing your pelvic muscles can help with symptoms, but if your rec-tocele is large, it may require surgical repair. The surgery involves reinforcing the fibrous connective tissue wall between the two organs to support your rectum and push it up and away from your vagina. Not only will your bloating improve, but having a bowel movement will be a lot easier, too.

Salt

Adding a lot of salt to your food can cause water retention, making you look and feel bloated. But food manufacturers often add salt to packaged food to preserve shelf life, so even if you put away your saltshaker, it can still be hard to avoid hidden caches of salt, especially if you eat a lot of processed or prepared food.

Solution

Don't add salt to your food, and check to see if spices and seasonings you're using have salt listed as one of the top ingredients (many do!). Read labels carefully to keep your salt intake in check, and aim for 1,000 milligrams or less per day to keep the bloat away.

82

Scar Tissue

If you've had abdominal or pelvic surgery (see "Surgery," page 181) or radiation to the area (see "Radiation," page 152), even if it was many years ago, you may have developed scar tissue that's causing you to bloat. Scar tissue creates cobweblike adhesions that can trap loops of bowel and cause a complete or partial bowel obstruction (see "Bowel Obstruction," page 31). If you have a complete obstruction as a result of scar tissue, you'll have severe pain, bloating, and maybe even vomiting as the segment of bowel above the blockage stretches and tries to push things through. If the blockage isn't relieved, your bowel can perforate (burst open), which is a medical emergency and can be fatal. If you have a partial bowel obstruction from scar tissue, you may also experience abdominal pain, but it will be less intense than with a complete obstruction, and chronic bloating will be your main complaint.

Solution

If you think scar tissue may be the cause of your bloating, you should have a medical evaluation that includes an X-ray or CAT (computerized axial tomography) scan of your abdomen to rule out a blockage or mass. The tests don't usually show the actual scar tissue, but they may reveal air-filled, dilated loops of bowel that suggest the presence of adhesions. If you're having recurrent episodes of obstruction, surgical exploration of your abdomen to look for and remove scar tissue is usually the next step. Milder obstructive symptoms can be treated with bowel rest or a liquid diet until things start moving again. The presence of scar tissue is one of the few exceptions to my "eat more fiber" rule, since a low-residue diet that limits fiber often leads to fewer episodes of obstruction.

83

Sedentary Lifestyle

If you're not moving, neither are your bowels! A sedentary lifestyle is a major contributor to slow transit through your gastrointestinal (GI) tract, which means bloating tends to be epidemic in places such as nursing homes and other chronic care facilities where the residents get little or no exercise. Sitting is the new smoking as far as your health is concerned, and that's especially true for your GI tract, where sitting at a computer all day can slow your transit to a crawl.

Solution

Regular exercise is important to stimulate peristalsis and keep your products of digestion moving efficiently through your gut. You don't have to run a marathon; even a walk around the block can help, and twisting yoga poses are especially good for dispersing gas pockets and moving things along. If your work involves sitting at a desk most of the day, set an alarm to go off every half hour as a reminder to get up and move around.

84

Sexually Transmitted Diseases

Sexually transmitted diseases such as chlamydia and gonor-rhea can cause infection of your reproductive organs (uterus, Fallopian tubes, ovaries), resulting in pelvic inflammatory disease (see "Pelvic Inflammatory Disease," page 146). If your bloating is accompanied by fever, pain, tenderness in the pelvic area, and a vaginal discharge, you may have pelvic inflammatory disease (PID) and you should get checked for sexually transmitted diseases right away.

Solution

A thorough pelvic exam with cultures and appropriate treatment (usually antibiotics) are essential if you have a sexually transmitted disease, because untreated PID can lead to infertility and ectopic pregnancies—a potentially life-threatening pregnancy that implants and grows in your Fallopian tubes rather than in your uterus. Safe sex techniques using barrier methods such as latex condoms can protect you from sexually transmitted diseases, which is a lot simpler than treating one once you have it.

85

Small Intestinal Bacterial Overgrowth*

Your small intestine is hardly sterile, but it has a lot less bacteria than your colon, the main living quarters for your gut bacteria. Small intestinal bacterial overgrowth (SIBO) is really just another term for dysbiosis that occurs when large amounts of not-so-good bacteria take up residence in your small intestine, causing gas, bloating, abdominal discomfort, and sometimes diarrhea or constipation. Nutritional deficiencies can also be part of the clinical presentation of SIBO, since your gut bacteria can affect the absorption of nutrients or consume them themselves. Antibiotic use is a major cause of SIBO, but impaired bowel motility and partial bowel obstruction that result in stasis (i.e., slowing down or stopping the movement) of your intestinal contents, and acid suppression that creates a hospitable environment for bacteria to overgrow, are also risk factors.

* See also "Dysbiosis," page 69.

We can test for SIBO by giving you a poorly absorbed sugar to eat that gets fermented by gut bacteria in your intestines. High levels of undesirable bacteria produce greater-than-expected levels of methane and hydrogen gases, which are expelled through your lungs and measured in your breath (via a lactulose or hydrogen breath test). Although breath tests can be useful, they're not always reliable, and a clinical diagnosis of SIBO based on history, physical exam, and signs and symptoms can be just as helpful.

Solution

Some physicians treat SIBO with an oral antibiotic called rifaximin (also known as Xifaxan) with the belief that, because rifaximin has activity against a lot of the bacteria that are overgrowing in the small intestine, using it to reduce their populations should lead to an improvement in symptoms. And it frequently does. The problem is that rifaximin, like all antibiotics, also acts against essential bacteria in the small intestine and colon and reduces those populations, too. The result is an initial improvement, which is almost always followed by relapse a few months later.

I recommend the same three-pronged approach to treat SIBO that we use for dysbiosis: *avoidance, encouragement,* and *repopulation.*

Avoid medications, foods, and other substances that contribute to the problem, including: antibiotics, acid suppressors, alcohol, artificial sweeteners, birth control pills, hormone replacement therapy, nonsteroidal anti-inflammatory drugs, steroids, and foods high in sugar and fat.

Encourage the growth of good bacteria by consuming foods with prebiotic ingredients that can increase your population of essential gut bacteria, including inulin, a naturally occurring carbohydrate found in plants such as artichokes, chicory, and jicama. Oats, dandelion greens, garlic, leeks, onions, and asparagus also contain prebiotics, especially when consumed raw. Fermented foods, such as sauerkraut, cabbage, and kefir, contribute to the growth of good bacteria and provide live bacteria themselves as a result of the fermentation process.

Repopulate your gut with large amounts of live bacteria in the form of a robust probiotic. Probiotics are live strains of bacteria that can be taken in pill, powder, or liquid form. They aren't considered drugs, so they're not regulated or tested for safety or efficacy, and you may have to do some research to find out which particular type may be best for you.

Identifying and remediating the cause of your SIBO is an essential step in getting rid of your bloating. The three-pronged approach I outlined might take some time before results are apparent, but it offers the possibility of a real cure.

Smoking

Smoking is guaranteed to add to your bloat in three important ways: you end up inhaling and swallowing a lot of air when you smoke (see "Aerophagia," page 3); the toxins in cigarette smoke cause inflammation in the lining of your stomach and intestines, which makes you bloated and uncomfortable; and smoking kills off beneficial bacteria in your digestive tract, leading to overgrowth of bloat-causing bad bacteria. If less bloating isn't enough incentive to give up nicotine for good, then keep in mind that smoking also increases your risk of digestive issues such as heartburn, peptic ulcers, liver disease, Crohn's disease, colon polyps, pancreatitis, gallstones, and most gastrointestinal cancers.

Solution

Quitting smoking reverses most of the harmful effects on your digestive system and relieves your bloating. The balance between the factors that harm and protect your stomach and small intestine returns to normal within a few hours of your quitting smoking, and the negative effects of smoking on how your liver handles medications also disappear when you stop smoking. Not smoking can improve symptoms of many digestive diseases or keep them from getting worse. For example, if you have Crohn's disease and quit smoking, you'll have milder symptoms than someone with Crohn's disease who continues to smoke, and the same is true if you have aerophagia, where smoking can be the main cause of symptoms.

Whether you go cold turkey or gradually decrease the number of cigarettes is up to you, but quitting smoking for good is one of the most important things you can do for your overall health, and for your bloat!

87

Soda

No one would argue that soda is a health food or part of a nutritious diet, but you may not realize that it could be the main reason you're bloated. The sweeteners in soda are usually sugar, high fructose corn syrup, poorly absorbed carbohydrates such as maltodextrin, or artificial sweeteners. The high sugar content (almost 10 teaspoons in some brands!) creates bloating because it leads to dysbiosis—overgrowth of undesirable bacterial species and yeast, especially candida, which feed on sugar—not to mention the extra weight a daily soda can lead to: a whopping 54,750 calories a year, which equals fifteen pounds.

Some studies have shown that artificial sweeteners cause a spike in insulin—the hormone responsible for fat storage, diabetes, inflammation, and belly fat. Although billed as low-calorie, they can cause just as much weight gain as regular soda. Poorly absorbed (nonnutritive) carbohydrates and artificial sweeteners don't get broken down and digested in your small intestine, but they undergo a lot of fermentation by bacteria in your colon, leading to gas and bloating. If you drink soda regularly, your bloating could also be the result of undiagnosed fructose intolerance, since soda sweetened with fructose greatly contributes to those symptoms.

Solution

Getting rid of soda of any kind (regular or diet) can be super helpful for your bloating. Even an occasional soda still has a ton of chemicals and sugar in it, and absolutely no nutritional value. Get in the habit of drinking more water—at least a liter a day—by identifying convenient times to drink it and scheduling it into your day. It may be during your daily commute, or between dinner and bedtime when you're at home and the bathroom is nearby. When you need some flavor and plain water just won't do, add a splash of fruit juice to carbonated water for a spritzer if the bubbles don't bother you, or use flat water with a ratio of four parts water to one part juice. Use electrolyte-rich coconut water as a rehydration solution, but don't overdo it, since the sugar and calories can add up. Try a green juice or fruit and veggie smoothie for hydration plus lots of nutrients, and experiment with hot or cold caffeine-free herbal teas (sweetened with raw honey if desired) as an alternative to soda.

Soy

f you're lactose intolerant, a soy latte may seem like a good idea, but processed soy can be a big contributor to your bloat. In Asia, small amounts of unprocessed fermented soy such as miso, natto, and tempeh are touted for their health benefits, primarily for encouraging the growth of beneficial bacterial species. But large amounts of processed unfermented soy, as we use in the West in place of dairy or as filler in foods, can have the opposite result: estrogen-like effects, which contribute to bloating, weight gain, and symptoms of estrogen dominance. Additionally, soy can slow down thyroid function and trigger thyroid disease in some individuals, which is a major cause of bloating.

Solution

Eliminate processed soy products from your diet, including soy milk, tofu, soy yogurt, and soy cheeses. Use unflavored, unsweetened almond milk, coconut milk, rice milk, or hemp milk instead of soy milk. Avoid products containing soy protein isolate, a common filler in packaged food—the less packaged food you eat, the less you have to worry about hidden sources of soy.

89

Sports Drinks

Unlike soda, these drinks are marketed as being healthy and full of important electrolytes, but unless you're training for an Ironman triathlon, or trying to add to your bloat, you don't need the extra sodium and other salts. The sugar and other sweeteners in sports drinks have the same bad effect on you as soda, causing bacterial overgrowth, weight gain, and bloating. You may not pay as much attention to how many calories you're consuming when you have a sports drink because you're lured in by the health claims, but in many cases the calories you're consuming far exceed what you've burned at the gym, and these drinks are full of bloat-causing chemicals, too.

Solution

The best way to hydrate after a workout is with water. If you're worried about electrolytes, eat a banana or drink some unsweetened, unflavored coconut water, which is high in potassium.

Steroids

Steroids are used to combat almost every form of inflammation, but because of their extensive side effects and ability to suppress your immune system, they're also a major cause of dysbiosis, disability, and even death. They're a danger to your microbiome because they suppress friendly bacteria and allow fungal species and other undesirables to overgrow, which can lead to major bloating. A weakened immune system also makes you more prone to infection. Even steroid creams applied to your skin can be absorbed in sufficient amounts to cause side effects if they're used for long enough and in high enough concentrations.

Solution

Because they suppress your adrenal glands' production of your native steroid hormones, if you've been prescribed steroids, they need to be tapered slowly. Abrupt discontinuation can result in adrenal crisis where your body lacks enough steroid hormones for proper function—a medical emergency requiring large doses of intravenous steroids.

An anti-inflammatory diet that excludes known causes of inflammation such as alcohol, refined sugars, processed grains, unhealthy fats, and poor-quality animal protein and focuses on large amounts of fresh organic vegetables, fruits, and healthy fats can help heal inflammation, keep you off steroids, and get rid of your bloat.

91

Stomach Cancer

S tomach cancer is usually asymptomatic early on, or causes vague symptoms such as bloating and a feeling of fullness in your upper abdomen. Bloating that occurs with indigestion or heartburn can be an early warning sign. Like pancreatic cancer, stomach cancer may have already reached an advanced stage at diagnosis, in which case you'll likely have additional symptoms of weight loss, nausea, and abdominal pain.

Solution

Infection with the bacteria *Helicobacter pylori* (see *Helicobacter pylori*, page 97) is one of the most important risk factors for developing stomach cancer, so it's a good idea to be tested for *H. pylori* if you think you may be at risk. *H. pylori* affects more than half the world's population, but fortunately it causes stomach cancer in only a tiny percentage. Nitrates and nitrites in smoked and processed meats are also risk factors for stomach cancer, and, in a small number of patients, stomach cancer is genetic.

92

Stress

Of all the things that conspire to cause bloating and gastro-intestinal (GI) distress, stress is one of the most prevalent. Chances are you've had the sensation of butterflies in your stomach, nausea, or gas right before a big event. Stress can worsen virtually every digestive condition, and bloating is no exception. Stress disrupts the normal hormonal messages throughout your gut that are important for bowel regularity, and it can trigger the fight-or-flight response that diverts resources from your digestive tract: it increases stomach acid, shunts blood away from your intestines, decreases enzyme secretion, slows down stomach emptying, and speeds up colonic contractions—all of which can add up to some serious bloating. Stress also induces responses in your gut that can affect your immune system, including increased intestinal permeability associated with leaky gut and food allergies, greater susceptibility to inflammation and infection, and overgrowth of harmful bacteria. A change in diet, anxiety over using unfamiliar bathroom facilities, jet lag, or dehydration can also add to stress-induced bloating.

If you think you may be anxious or overly stressed, it's a good idea to have your mental health assessed by a professional, especially if you've been diagnosed with irritable bowel syndrome and told that stress is partly to blame. Researchers frequently make reference to the "second brain" in your gut—the millions of nerve cells in your digestive tract that allow you to "feel" the inner world of your gut. Your gut-brain interaction is essential for good digestive health. Not feeling well psychologically makes it much more challenging for you to have a healthy, bloat-free digestive tract.

Like many people, you may have a lot of stress in your life, and you may be really bloated. But could stress actually be causing your bloat? The answer is: it could be. There definitely seems to be a group of people whose bloating is entirely due to stress, although more commonly stress is an exacerbating factor, making symptoms worse.

Solution

If you think stress may be contributing to your GI symptoms but you're not sure, here are some useful signs and symptoms to look for:

PHYSICAL SYMPTOMS
- Stiff or tense muscles, especially in the neck or shoulders
- Headaches
- Shakiness or tremors
- Loss of interest in sex
- Weight gain or loss
- Restlessness

BEHAVIORAL SYMPTOMS

- Procrastination
- Grinding teeth
- Difficulty completing work assignments
- Changes in the amount of alcohol or food you consume
- Sleeping too much or too little

EMOTIONAL SYMPTOMS

- Crying
- Overwhelming sense of tension or pressure
- Trouble relaxing
- Nervousness
- Quick temper
- Depression
- Poor concentration
- Trouble remembering things
- Loss of sense of humor

Gut-directed hypnotherapy (GHT) to relieve stress is an effective therapy for GI distress and bloating, and it is found to be superior to medical treatment alone in clinical studies. Quality-of-life outcomes are improved and GHT has a long-term positive effect even in difficult-to-treat cases of stress-induced bloating. The practice involves getting your mind and body into a deep state of relaxation with the help of a trained therapist, who then makes positive comments about the state of your digestive tract and your ability to control symptoms. Most biofeedback practitioners practice GHT, as do many classically trained psychologists and licensed clinical social workers.

93

Sugar

If you're like most Americans, you probably consume close to your body weight in sugar every year. Sugars are carbohydrates made up of one (monosaccharide), two (disaccharide), or multiple (oligosaccharide) linked molecules. Glucose and fructose, found primarily in fruits, vegetables, and industrial processed foods, and their slightly less sweet cousin, galactose, which is found primarily in dairy products and sugar beets, are simple monosaccharide sugars. Sucrose, also known as table sugar, is a disaccharide of glucose and fructose. Lactose is a disaccharide of glucose and galactose that occurs naturally in milk.

Your sweet tooth may be playing a major role in your bloating through a number of different mechanisms, including micronutrient deficiencies, inflammation, bacterial imbalance, and yeast overgrowth. Because sugary foods often replace more nutritious ones and because sugar is devoid of the important nutrients your body needs to function well, overconsumption can lead to micronutrient deficiencies that have broad health implications, in addition to bloating. Diets high in sugar also contribute to inflammation throughout your body and immune suppression, both of which can lead to serious bloating.

Too much sugar sends gut bacteria into a feeding frenzy, resulting in overgrowth of lots of undesirable species whose waste products include bloat-forming gas. Excessive sugar consumption can also cause overgrowth of yeast species such as candida, which is associated with fatigue, leaky gut syndrome, and, of course, bloating. Finally, in a vicious cycle that is just plain unfair, bacterial imbalance and yeast overgrowth from excessive sugar consumption leads right back to intense cravings for more sugar!

Solution

Part of why sugar is so hard to quit is because it stimulates production of the neurotransmitter dopamine, which is associated with intense pleasure. Eating lots of sugary foods can create the same effect a drug addict experiences after taking cocaine or heroin—because the same dopamine receptors in your brain get stimulated. Here are some ways to decrease your sugar intake—and your bloat:

- Lots of people turn to a low-carb lifestyle to help them lose weight as well as lose cravings, but it's easy to overdo the bacon, eggs, and hamburger patties—not a great idea if you're concerned about things such as heart disease, cancer, and your overall health, and too much animal protein will make you constipated and bloated.

Don't eliminate healthy carbohydrates; instead, incor-
porate lots of vegetables and "slow carbs" that are high
in fiber, such as legumes, sweet potatoes, nuts, brown
rice, and quinoa.

- Cut out processed carbohydrates such as cake, cookies,
  ice cream, and candy.
- Cut out starchy foods such as bagels, pasta, bread, white
  potatoes, and white rice, which are just glucose molecules, arranged differently.
- Cut down on grapes, bananas, and sweet tropical fruit
  and eat more fibrous choices, such as apples, pears, and
  berries, which don't cause as much of a spike in your
  blood sugar but still provide lots of healthy fiber and
  nutrients.

94

Surgery

Forget about whether your C-section, hysterectomy, appendectomy, gallbladder removal, or any other surgery you've recently had was actually necessary (that's a whole other book!), and think about what you felt like after you had it. Chances are bloating was a big part of your post-op recovery. During laparoscopic (minimally invasive) surgery, carbon dioxide, nitrous oxide, or helium gases are pumped into your belly to help keep things inflated and improve visibility. The gases end up increasing your intra-abdominal pressure, which can mean massive bloating after surgery until the gases dissipate or are absorbed by your tissues.

You also get tons of IV fluids during surgery to counteract the effects of anesthesia and any blood or fluid losses that occur. Liters of extra fluid can leave you with extreme post-op puffiness and it may take weeks for your bloating to go down. After surgery you're usually immobilized on your back for a while, and receiving narcotic pain medications—both of which will slow down your bowels and conspire to bloat you even more. On the off chance you're still not massively bloated, antibiotics given during and after your surgery are likely to kill off droves of your healthy bacteria and leave you with an imbalanced bloat-promoting microbiome that may never fully recover.

Solution

The best rule of thumb for preventing post-op bloating is to avoid surgery unless absolutely necessary. Bloating is a common problem after surgery, but fortunately, it's not life-threatening. Given all the possible serious complications of surgery, including bleeding, infection, stroke, heart attack, blood clots, pulmonary embolism, bowel perforation, respiratory arrest, and possibly death, it's critical to make sure that you really need whatever surgery you're about to have. Assuming you do, then getting up and out of bed and walking laps around the nurses' station as soon as it's physically safe to do so, minimizing your use of narcotic pain medication, asking if antibiotics can be withheld unless there's an actual infection, and drinking liquids as soon as you're allowed so they don't have to give you as much IV fluids are all great post-op bloat-busting strategies—plus a little prune juice, which can go a long way for surgery-induced backup!

95

Thyroid Problems

Hormones are chemical messengers that are made in your glands, released into your bloodstream, and then travel to millions of cells in your body, telling them what to do. The thyroid gland (located in your neck at around the level of your Adam's apple) makes thyroid hormones that control your metabolism. If your body were an airport, your thyroid gland would be air traffic control, secreting tiny bursts of hormone here and there to rev up your metabolism when your body needs a boost and dampening production when you're at rest and need a little less.

An underactive thyroid gland (hypothyroidism) slows down a lot of your bodily functions, including lymphatic drainage, leading to fluid retention and excess water weight. This causes a puffy feeling all over, particularly in your abdominal area, which is why bloating is so common if you have thyroid problems. Hypothyroidism can also cause bloating by slowing down transit through your colon. Even if you're on thyroid replacement therapy, the bloating and puffiness often remain because a pill taken once a day can't replicate the minute-to-minute adjustments in hormone secretion a well-functioning thyroid gland is constantly making.

If you're a woman over thirty, your risk of developing a thyroid problem is almost 25 percent. The high sensitivity of the tests used is one explanation for that impressive number, but thyroid disease is definitely on the rise because of chemicals in our environment that act as endocrine disruptors and throw our glands out of whack, and because of nutritional deficiencies such as not getting enough iodine and consuming too much processed soy, which affect the function of your thyroid and ultimately make you more bloated.

Solution

If you suspect that a poorly functioning thyroid gland may be to blame for your bloating, it's important to know that not all cases of thyroid dysfunction can be accurately diagnosed by a blood test. Your thyroid hormone levels may be within the normal range for the lab but not for your body. Since there's also a lot of debate about what constitutes a normal result with the existing tests, it may be helpful to see a specialist with experience in treating borderline thyroid dysfunction rather than initiating self-treatment with over-the-counter remedies, which, like prescription thyroid replacement therapy, can lead to unwanted side effects if taken unnecessarily. Removing irritants such as soy, gluten, and dairy from your diet can help improve your thyroid function (and your bloating), even if you've been diagnosed with an underactive thyroid.

96

Ulcerative Colitis*

Ulcerative colitis (UC) is an autoimmune disease where your body wages war against its own healthy tissues, leading to inflammation in your colon. Bloody diarrhea is the hallmark of UC, often accompanied by bloating because of all the ulceration and inflammation. UC can also cause symptoms outside your gastrointestinal tract, including joint pain, fever, kidney stones, skin lesions, fatigue, and mouth ulcers. More and more we're recognizing that alterations in the microbiome play a causative role in autoimmune diseases such as UC and are looking at treatment options that include restoring gut bacteria to a healthy balance.

Solution

Dietary modifications that remove pro-inflammatory foods such as refined sugar, processed grains, dairy, gluten, and unhealthy fats, along with a robust probiotic (live bacteria) supplement in

* See also "Crohn's Disease," page 56.

conjunction with medications of low toxicity if needed, is the most holistic approach to treating UC, although some practitioners (and patients) opt for medical therapy alone, without relying on diet and lifestyle changes.

Biofeedback, which can teach you how to relieve spasm in the muscles of your digestive tract through mind-body techniques, and acupuncture, which can lead to an overall relaxed state, can also be very helpful in controlling bloating and other symptoms of UC. If diet and lifestyle changes don't help, then stronger drugs that are more efficacious but also have more side effects are usually the next step. For most people, there really is no downside to using food as medicine, and there are clearly countless other benefits to eating a healthy diet besides putting your UC into remission. But if your disease is really severe, you may need to cool things down with stronger conventional therapy first before embarking on the slower pace of dietary change, probiotics, and mind-body techniques.

97

Urinary Tract Infections

I f you think your bloating may be because you have a urinary tract infection (UTI), the first order of business is to make sure you really have one. Bladder irritation from interstitial cystitis, or from endometriosis, fibroids, diverticulosis, or a full colon pressing on your bladder can mimic all the signs and symptoms of a UTI, including urinary urgency, frequency, burning, pelvic pain, and, of course, bloating. Many practitioners have gotten into the habit of treating first and asking questions later, and some don't even bother to send a urine specimen for analysis and culture. Lots of white blood cells found on urinalysis may indicate infection, but it should be confirmed with a urine culture that shows more than one hundred thousand colony-forming units (CFUs) on a "clean-catch" urine specimen (i.e., obtained midstream).

Taking lots of antibiotics, even for culture-proven UTIs, can put you at risk for more infections by reducing your population of beneficial bacteria, allowing undesirable species to overgrow and become more resistant and aggressive. When these patho-genic gut bacteria (usually *E. coli*) accidentally stray into the vicinity of your bladder, as can happen from time to time, they can cause more UTIs and bloating, so you need to be judicious in deciding whether to treat your urinary symptoms with an antibiotic.

Solution

Even though UTIs can be overdiagnosed, there are some circumstances where you don't want to allow a UTI to go undiagnosed or untreated. Fever, chills, or flank pain may indicate an upper UTI involving your kidneys (pyelonephritis), for which you should seek immediate medical care. For more minor symptoms, here are some ideas to help prevent UTIs and relieve symptoms:

- Hydrate, hydrate, and hydrate some more to flush your urinary system. Aim for at least eight 8-ounce glasses of water daily.
- Take D-mannose, a naturally occurring substance found in cranberries that helps prevent *E. coli* bacteria from sticking to the wall of your bladder and setting up shop. Take 1 teaspoon or 2 grams, four times a day, for five days. D-mannose can also be taken prophylactically, that is, to prevent infection if you're prone to UTIs.
- Empty your bladder frequently, especially after intercourse.
- Wipe front to back after bowel movements, because most UTIs are caused by bacteria from your colon that gain entrance to your urinary system.

98

Uterine Cancer

Bloating plus abnormal vaginal bleeding can be a sign of uterine cancer that develops from cells in the lining of your uterus. Other symptoms include a watery or blood-tinged vaginal discharge, pelvic pain, or pain with intercourse or urination, but sometimes bloating, a change in bowel habits, and the new onset of constipation are the only initial signs. Important risk factors for developing uterine cancer include using estrogen supplements (that don't also contain progesterone), taking tamoxifen for breast cancer, a history of radiation therapy, a family history of uterine cancer, or a family history of a form of inherited colon cancer called Lynch syndrome.

Solution

How do you know if your bloating isn't just a nuisance but a sign of something more worrisome, like uterine cancer? Certain combinations of symptoms, in the right setting, especially if you have a strong family history or additional risk factors, may point to a more serious diagnosis that needs further investigation. Fortunately, even aggressive cancers, when caught early enough, can be treated and often cured. If you have any concerns at all about whether your bloating may represent something more than just a bothersome symptom, don't hesitate to seek a thorough evaluation.

99

Wheat Allergy

Wheat allergies are fairly common, especially in children, and bloating can be one of the symptoms. If you have a wheat allergy, your immune system will react to wheat by making immunoglobulin E antibodies, which can be measured by a blood test. A wheat allergy can also be diagnosed by injecting wheat under your skin. Bumps, redness, and irritation that occur within about fifteen minutes signify a positive test, although even with a positive test, you may not necessarily have symptoms when you eat wheat.

Solution

If you have a wheat allergy and experience bloating or other allergic symptoms when you eat wheat, then you should avoid it. If you don't experience symptoms, then you can have it.

100

Yeast Overgrowth[*]

Yeast (fungal) overgrowth can cause an itchy vaginal discharge, but it may also be the cause of your bloat. When you take antibiotics, large amounts of good bacteria are destroyed along with whatever bad bacteria you're trying to get rid of, and yeast species quickly overgrow to fill the void. Yeast grows in damp places, such as under your arms, in your groin, in your mouth, and in your gut, where they're involved in fermenting food, a process that produces carbon dioxide gas—and lots of bloat! An overabundance of yeast in your intestines can damage the lining of your gut, resulting in poor absorption of nutrients and a condition called leaky gut (see "Leaky Gut," page 118), which is also a major cause of bloating.

Additional signs and symptoms of yeast overgrowth include:

- Depression
- Fatigue
- Food cravings

[*] See also "Candida," page 36.

- Food sensitivities
- Headaches
- Impaired concentration
- Nail infections
- Rectal itching
- Skin problems such as eczema, acne, hives, athlete's foot, ringworm, and dandruff
- Thrush (white lesions in the mouth)
- Unstable blood sugar

Solution

If you have yeast overgrowth, you may be tempted to go on a search-and-destroy mission and treat it with lots of heavy-duty antifungals. But rebalancing your microbiome with essential bacteria that can crowd out yeast and keep their growth in check is the hallmark of a successful anti-yeast treatment program, not just suppression with medication. Eating lots of indigestible plant fiber to feed your good bacteria, avoiding sugary, starchy foods that attract yeast, and taking a good probiotic can make all the difference for yeast-induced bloating.

Z-Pak*

A Z-Pak refers to a short course of the antibiotic Zithromax (azithromycin), usually given for three to five days for respiratory, skin, or ear infections, or for sexually transmitted diseases. Even though only taken for a few days, just as with other antibiotics, the effects of a Z-Pak on your population of healthy gut bacteria can be devastating, and bloating and diarrhea are common side effects.

Solution

If you've been prescribed a Z-Pak for a non–life threatening infection, it's essential to figure out whether you really need it or not, because although some of the side effects (such as diarrhea and nausea) may disappear within a few days, it may take months to recover from the damage to your microbiome and the chronic bloating that accompanies it. Ask your doctor whether what

---

* See also "Antibiotics," page 13.

you're being treated for might resolve on its own and if watchful waiting is an option. If you do end up having to take a Z-Pak, it's still possible to mitigate the damage by supporting your gut and your microbes during and after. These tips will help minimize microbial loss, encourage rapid regrowth, and alleviate your bloating:

1. Take a probiotic during and after the Z-Pak. Several studies have documented the usefulness of probiotics in decreasing side effects such as antibiotic-associated diarrhea (AAD), as well as repopulating the gut. You should start the probiotic at the same time you start the Z-Pak, and continue it for at least one month after finishing the Z-Pak. Probiotics containing various strains of *Lactobacillus* and *Bifidobacterium* are the most useful.

2. Eat prebiotic foods to support your microbiome. Foods high in fiber and resistant starch are especially important when you're taking a Z-Pak. Not only do they provide food for your microbes, but they also help to promote species diversity, which can decrease dramatically after a course of antibiotics. Fermented foods such as sauerkraut and kimchi feed your gut bacteria as well as provide additional live microbes themselves.

3. Eliminate sugary, starchy foods. Omitting these foods from your diet is important when you're taking a Z-Pak. Foods (and drinks) high in sugar and starchy foods that are broken down into simple sugars in the gut send undesirable yeast species into a feeding frenzy, further contributing to microbial imbalance induced

by the antibiotics. If you're prone to yeast infections, following a strict anti-yeast diet that excludes any and all sugar while taking a Z-Pak—and for thirty days afterward—may be advisable.

4. Drink ginger tea. Ginger has a soothing effect on the digestive system and can help to reduce gas and bloating associated with taking a Z-Pak. For best results, peel a one-inch piece of fresh gingerroot, cut it into small pieces, and place in a teapot or thermal carafe. Then add two cups of boiling water and let steep for twenty to thirty minutes. Strain and serve.

Index

Boldface page number range indicates a chapter about a term.

ALSO BY ROBYNNE CHUTKAN, M.D.

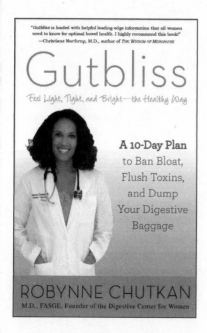

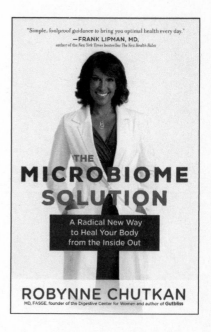

A complete guide to good gastrointestinal health for women, with a ten-day digestive tune-up.

Distills the latest microbiome research into a practical program for boosting overall health.

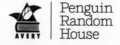